ARTICULATION
AND
LEARNING

ARTICULATION
— AND —
LEARNING

NEW DIMENSIONS IN RESEARCH, DIAGNOSTICS, AND THERAPY

Edited by

W. DEAN WOLFE

Associate Professor and Director
Speech Clinic
Oberlin College
Oberlin, Ohio

and

DANIEL J. GOULDING

Associate Professor and Chairman
Department of Communication Studies
Oberlin College
Oberlin, Ohio

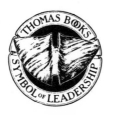

CHARLES C THOMAS • PUBLISHER
Springfield • Illinois • U.S.A.

Published and Distributed Throughout the World by

CHARLES C THOMAS • PUBLISHER

Bannerstone House

301-327 East Lawrence Avenue, Springfield, Illinois, U.S.A.

© *1973, by* CHARLES C THOMAS • PUBLISHER

ISBN 0-398-02702-1

Library of Congress Catalog Card Number: 72-88493

*With THOMAS BOOKS careful attention is given to all details of
manufacturing and design. It is the Publisher's desire to present books that are
satisfactory as to their physical qualities and artistic possibilities and
appropriate for their particular use. THOMAS BOOKS will be true to those
laws of quality that assure a good name and good will.*

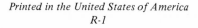
Printed in the United States of America

R-1

CONTRIBUTORS

LESTER F. AUNGST, Ph.D.

Assistant Professor and
Associate Director of Training
Speech and Hearing Center
Temple University
Philadelphia, Pennsylvania

EDGAR R. GARRETT, Ph.D.

Professor and Head
Department of Speech and
Assistant Dean in Arts and Sciences
New Mexico State University
Las Cruces, New Mexico

FRANCIS A. GRIFFITH, Ph.D.

Associate Professor of Speech Pathology and Audiology
Memphis State University
Memphis, Tennessee

KATHERINE S. HARRIS, Ph.D.

Research Associate
Haskins Laboratories and
Professor of Speech
City University of New York
New York, New York

JOHN V. IRWIN, Ph.D.

Pope M. Farrington Professor
Department of Audiology and Speech Pathology
Memphis State University
Memphis, Tennessee

EUGENE T. MCDONALD, Ed.D.

Research Professor in Speech Pathology
The Pennsylvania State University
State College, Pennsylvania

ROBERT L. MILISEN, Ph.D.

Professor of Speech Pathology
Indiana University
Bloomington, Indiana

DONALD E. MOWRER, Ph.D.

Associate Professor of Speech
Arizona State University
Tempe, Arizona

ROBERT L. RINGEL, Ph.D.

Professor and Head
Department of Audiology and Speech Sciences
Purdue University
Lafayette, Indiana

WILLIAM H. TEDFORD, JR., Ph.D.

Associate Professor of Psychology
Southern Methodist University
Dallas, Texas

MILDRED C. TEMPLIN, Ph.D.

Professor of Child Psychology
University of Minnesota
Minneapolis, Minnesota

LAWRENCE J. TURTON, Ph.D.

Program Director for Speech and
Language Pathology
Institute for the Study of Mental Retardation
University of Michigan
Ann Arbor, Michigan

HARRIS WINITZ, Ph.D.

Associate Professor of Speech
University of Missouri at Kansas City
Kansas City, Missouri

PREFACE

DEFECTIVE articulation is often assumed to be a relatively uncomplicated problem in speech communication requiring relatively simple procedures for correction. Moreover, clinicians often appear to assume that knowledge of the nature of speech articulation and its defects is complete and well defined. As with most seemingly simple processes of communication behavior, however, research into the nature of articulatory acquisition and its defects continues to reveal new dimensions, complexities and unexplored terrain. Indeed, the intrusion of a proliferating number of new theoretical constructs, research findings and clinical procedures into this previously quiet and relatively secure area of speech pathology has confronted the conscientious practicing clinician as well as the newly interested student with a fecund but scattered and sometimes conflicting body of literature.

It is the purpose of this book to bring into critical relationship these new and diverse perspectives and to accentuate the latest developments in research, diagnostics and therapy. New theoretical concepts and research findings are presented by recognized scholars who are frequently the originators of the perspectives and procedures discussed. While considerable emphasis in the book is upon recent application of behavioral models and learning theory paradigms to an understanding of articulatory acquisition and to the clinical management of articulation disorders, such emphasis is developed with reference to previous research findings, and to pertinent neurophysiological, linguistic and psychological dimensions.

In order to achieve a coherent presentation of such diverse materials and perspectives for the newly interested student and to enhance the value of the book as a reference source for the practicing clinician, the chapters are arranged in a continuum from those which emphasize scientific and theoretical foundations to those which emphasize clinically oriented research.

In presenting a substantive introduction to the foundations of articulatory acquisition and behavior, the first four chapters written respectively by Harris, Ringel, Templin and Tedford provide a critical review of previous research and a discussion of current findings in the neurophysiology of articulation, oral sensation and perception, developmental aspects of articulation learning and the potential applications of verbal learning theory and research findings to the study of articulation.

Chapter 5 by Winitz emphasizes behavioral and linguistic relationships in speech modification, and Chapter 6 by Garrett reports and discusses findings of experimental research in the use of automated and programmed therapies: these two chapters provide a natural transition from the basic research emphases of the opening chapters to the clinical orientation of the final chapters.

In the chapters which deal specifically with clinical research in the management of articulation disorders, Mowrer (Chapter 7) presents a case for the use of recently developed operant procedures in articulation therapy, Irwin and Griffith (Chapter 8) present a study of the paired-stimuli technique in articulatory modification, Turton (Chapter 9) explores and emphasizes important relationships between diagnostic and therapeutic procedures and Aungst and McDonald (Chapter 10) examine the problem of evaluating clinical effectiveness.

In the final chapter, Milisen undertakes the somewhat olympian task of moving the reader toward an integrated understanding of the diverse options and procedures available to the clinician in the treatment of articulation disorders. He proposes a rationale for harmonizing the potential for clinical artistry with the demands for rational and scientifically based procedures of treatment. In the course of developing his perspectives, Milisen provides an effective summary and conclusion to the book.

While it is obviously not possible to explore all major dimensions of articulation learning in depth within the scope of a single volume, the present work provides a valuable current review of important theoretical and clinical developments, some new dimensions in the study of articulation and reveals a number of areas in need of further research.

The editors wish to acknowledge that the original stimulus for this book was provided by a special study institute on articulation and learning held at Oberlin College in the summer of 1969 and funded by a grant from the Bureau of Education for the Handicapped, United States Office of Education, under Public Law 85–926. We are grateful to the forty participating speech clinicians from throughout the country and to the contributing scholars at the conference, whose questions, discussions and presentations not only revealed the need for a book of this kind, but indicated a number of areas requiring attention. We are particularly grateful to Dr. Richard Schiefelbusch for his encouragement and support of the project in its initial planning stages.

We are also indebted to the Oberlin College Stenographic Service for its help in preparing the manuscript; to the typist, Richard Hope; and to Carolyn Husted for secretarial assistance.

W. D. W.

D. J. G.

CONTENTS

ARTICULATION
AND
LEARNING

CHAPTER I

THE PHYSIOLOGICAL SUBSTRATE OF SPEAKING

KATHERINE S. HARRIS

W HEN someone speaks and someone else listens, the listener performs the difficult task of extracting a message from an extremely complex acoustic signal. This task is performed so effortlessly by the normal adult listener that it is difficult for him to understand that there is any problem in doing it. However, if we compare the signal and the message extracted, it becomes easier to understand the magnitude of the listener's accomplishment. This chapter will summarize what we know about the production of the speech signal, the relationship between the acoustic signal and the mechanism which produced it.

There are three quite different types of problems for a listener in comprehending a speaker's message. First, the speech signal is different acoustically, depending on the size and shape of the vocal tract which produces it. These effects are quite well understood (see, for example, Stevens and House, 1961), and it is possible to normalize the acoustic signal (Fujisaki and Nakamura, 1969) by mathematical techniques. Apparently, the listener performs some such normalization, and infers the gesture which produces a given speech sound, regardless of whether the speaker is a child or an adult.

A second type of analysis which the listener appears to perform is to disentangle, in perception, the aspects of the acoustic signal which have to do with what have been called source characteristics

NOTE: The research upon which this chapter is based was supported in part by a grant from the National Institute of Dental Research.

and signal characteristics. Roughly speaking, this division has a physiologic parallel. The *source* characteristics can be referred back to the action of the larynx and the lungs, while the *signal* characteristics can be referred to the upper articulators.

A third type of analysis which the listener appears to make can be described as *segmenting*. Virtually all systems of analysis of spoken messages describe them as made up of a limited number of elements, which are recombined and strung out. However, analysis of any physiological measure of speech production shows a continuous flow of activity without any clear units. It is unclear how the listener makes the division into units or on what principles.

This chapter will attempt to summarize what we know about the physiological base on which the listener operates.

PHYSIOLOGICAL TECHNIQUES IN SPEECH RESEARCH

Physiological studies have been conducted with either of two kinds of general techniques: one kind, which we might call viewing techniques, includes use of pulsed ultrasound, endoscopic movies, cinefluorography, and photography of the lips and jaw. In these studies, the measures taken are related to the movement of one or several articulatory structures directly. The advantage of such techniques is that, since the acoustic speech wave is determined by vocal tract shape, such measures are close to what the listener hears.

Recent advances in viewing techniques are summarized in a series of articles in an ASHA special report — particularly by Bzoch (1970) on x-ray and cineradiography, by Harris (1970) on endoscopy and by Lubker (1970) on a closely related technique, the use of pulsed ultrasound.

A second kind of technique, electromyography, has the advantage of being one step closer to central speech processing. Furthermore, in one sense, electromyographic measures are simpler than shape measures, since they reflect the action patterns — unhindered by mechanical linkages — that are sent down to the articulators. However, signal size varies in a complex way with the speed and distance-to-target of articulator movement, and so includes context effects which are not directly represented in articulator movement (MacNeilage, 1970; Ohman, Leandersson, and Persson, 1966). Recent advances in electromyographic measurement technique have been reviewed by Harris (1970), by Gay and Harris (1971) and by Hirano and Ohala (1969).

THE PHYSIOLOGICAL SUBSTRATE OF SEGMENTAL PLACE-OF-ARTICULATION GESTURES

Fairly clear physiological divisions correspond to the linguistic distinction between segmental and suprasegmental phones. In general, information about segmental place gestures is conveyed by the shape of the upper vocal tract. Recent work has had two somewhat different focuses of interest — descriptive studies of shape and its muscular determinants and theoretical studies which attempt to account for the general organization of the speech process.

Descriptive Studies

Classical description of upper vocal tract shape for vowels has been organized around the two dimensions of tongue height and back-front position of the place of maximum constriction of the tongue. Recent cinefluorographic work (Perkell, 1969; Ladefoged, deClerk and Harshman, 1971) has provided us with a fairly complete description of these aspects of vocal tract shape for various vowels. However, a given tongue height is not related to a unique position of the articulators, as Lindblom and Sundberg (1971) have recently pointed out. It is determined by jaw opening and tongue humping, acting jointly. Furthermore, they showed that if speakers were asked to produce a given vowel with the jaws propped open by blocks, they were able to compensate for jaw position change by tongue adjustment. This suggests that the memory storage for vowels is in terms of a mouth target position rather than as a fixed muscle configuration. Individual speakers may, however, have preferred paths to the attainment of a given articulator position. Raphael (1971) has shown that two different speakers may use a different balance of jaw opening and tongue fronting to distinguish between the tense-lax vowel pairs /i–I/ and /e–ɛ/.

For the consonants, information at a descriptive level varies a great deal depending on the place of articulation of the consonant. The movement of the lips for the bilabial consonant has, of course, been studied in greatest detail, since the structures themselves are readily available for direct viewing, and the underlying musculature is not difficult to tap (Ohman, Leandersson and Persson, 1967a; Fromkin, 1966; Harris, Lysaught and Schvey, 1965). At the level of cinefluorographic viewing, velar and alveolar consonants have been described by Perkell (1969). However, the underlying muscular description is fragmentary for velar consonants, and nonexistent for alveolar consonants. The reason for this is that fine shaping, especially of the tongue tip, appears to be controlled largely by the intrinsic tongue muscles. As yet, techniques have not been developed for studying these muscles.

The determinants of upper vocal tract shape are, of course, the muscles which act on the jaw, on the hyoid bone, on the pharynx, and on the tongue itself. Although inferences about the function of the various muscles, on the basis of gross anatomy, have been discussed for some time (Van Riper and Irwin, 1958; Ladefoged, deClerk and Harshman, 1971), direct recording from most of them has been possible only in the last few years, since the development of hooked wire electrodes. At present, mapping studies are available only on a few of this large series. It has been shown that jaw opening in speech is controlled by a complex interaction of two of the suprahyoid muscles — the anterior belly of the digastric and the geniohyoid (Harris, 1971) and the strap muscles of the neck (Ohala and Hirose, 1970). The mylohyoid muscle, sometimes described as a jaw depressor in the chewing literature (Mohler, 1966), appears to function in speech to raise and back the tongue (Smith, 1970; Harris, 1971).

The action of muscles which act on the tongue directly to position it in the back-front dimension is even less well understood. The genioglossus clearly acts to raise and front the tongue (Smith, 1970; Raphael, 1971; Harris, 1971). The pharyngeal constrictors act to back the tongue (Smith, 1970; Berti, 1971) and the palatoglossus is associated with tongue backing and raising (Berti, 1971). Two other muscles of the velopharyngeal port are associated with backing and raising because of their effects on pharyngeal size directly — the levator palatini and palatopharyngeus (Berti, 1971; Lubker, Fritzell and Lindquist, 1971).

The Organization of Segmental Place Units

As stated above, one of the central problems at the level of speech production is how to rationalize the observation that, while language is heard as a succession of unitary sounds drawn from a small set and organized into many combinations, the acoustic form of language does not show clearly the same organization, nor do the articulatory gestures that produce the sounds. Thus, segments that are heard as the same speech sound show large variations of acoustic form, depending on context; moreover, the segments are so entangled with each other at the acoustic level that it is usually not possible to separate, or segment, them. Likewise, the gestures associated with individual speech sounds vary with context and merge into adjacent gestures to give an unsegmentable whole. How, then, is one to identify the segmental units of sound and account for their interactions with each other and their organization into larger units? And, in articulatory terms, what are the unitary events of articulation, how can they be characterized, and how are they organized into the larger gestures of syllable, word, and breath-group?

These questions about units and hierarchical organization can, of course, be approached either from above or below. Chomsky and Halle (1968) have made a major effort to extend a linquistic rule-based account all the way down to the string of phonetic segments that lie just above overt speech. The approach from below, by way of phonetic description, starts with observations of language as it is produced by native speakers and attempts to infer from these data a linguistic structure that will meet the dual tests of simplicity and adequacy in accounting for the observations. These various approaches, linguistic from above and phonetic from below, have converged to an uneasy meeting at about the level of phonology: the features and phonetic segments of the one do not quite match onto the segments and features inferred by the other from observation and experimentation. It may be that additional information about muscle activities and resulting configurations will clarify the relationship of actual speech gestures to linguistic descriptions. In any case, the theoretical formulations can guide the experimentalist to significant problems.

In considering the varied forms in which a particular speech sound may occur, it is useful to distinguish between two general kinds of allophonic variation: extrinsic and intrinsic. Extrinsic allophones (such as light and dark /l/ in English) are optional, i.e. not an automatic consequence of articulatory constraints, and may serve as a single phoneme in one language, or as more than one in another. Intrinsic allophones, on the other hand, are presumed to be universal and arise from some property of the speech mechanism. Indeed, it has been suggested by Fromkin (1970) that when a speech error of the slip-of-the-tongue variety occurs it will have, in articulation, appropriate characteristics for its slipped position. This would imply some low-level characteristics of allophonic variation which are separated from some higher level of planning. One way of describing these characteristics is to assume that each phoneme is stored as a fixed articulatory position, or target (MacNeilage, 1970). This target is not always attained when one speaks, but failures of attainment are a consequence of the way the articulatory system operates — that is, failures of attainment can be ascribed to such things as the sluggishness of the articulators in responding to commands and to a lack of perfect synchronization among all the articulatory components of a given phone (Lisker, 1970). Indeed there is good evidence that the listener assembles information about a single phone from parts of the acoustic wave that are not necessarily concurrent (Liberman, 1970).

Studies of allophonic variation can be made by acoustic-perceptual means as well as by direct physiological methods. Thus, both Lindblom (1963) and Ohman (1967b) have used acoustic data to make inferences about the nature of the differences in vocal tract shape between allophones. This procedure works because the acoustic theory of speech production (Fant, 1960; Stevens and House, 1961) will often, in practice, allow direct inference from acoustic output back to shape, at least for certain contexts and a single speaker.

Different types of allophonic variation have been found and studied in two rather different circumstances: one is the failure of vowels to reach a stable position when they are not stressed, or when speaking rate is increased, and is usually described as vowel reduction or undershoot; the other is the variation in articulation of a phone depending on its phonetic context and is often referred to as coarticulation.

A careful study of vowel reduction, using acoustic data, was made by Lindblom (1963). He had subjects produce CVC syllables in a sentence frame such that the stress on the syllable varied and, in consequence, the duration of the vowel varied. He then found that the shorter the vowel, the farther from target frequencies (and, by inference, from a single articulatory shape) the vowel formants fell. Lindblom was able to show that this failure to attain the vowel target could be predicted from a simple model in which there is presumed to be an activating command for each phoneme element; however, due to the inertia of the articulatory structures, there is a time delay between the arrival of the command and the completion of movement. Then, when successive commands are too closely spaced, the moving articulators will not have had time to attain target positions.

Lindblom's undershoot model implies systematic departures from the attainment of constant articulator target position as a function of stress or rate of articulation. Such departures have been demonstrated at the level of articulator movement by Houde (1967), who measured tongue position as a function of stress variation in a cineradiographic study. However, Lindblom supposes that these effects are due solely to mechanical factors, i.e. the sluggishness of the articulators; consequently, electromyographic signal size should be invariant over changes in stress, though the temporal spacing between signals for different parts of the utterance will alter. A preliminary study (Harris, Gay, Sholes and Lieberman, 1968) failed to support this model. A comparison of the amplitude of electromyographic signals for consonants in heavily emphasized words (in sentences) with analogous signals for the same words unemphasized, shows that consonant amplitudes for the stressed words were somewhat greater than for the unstressed.

More recently (Harris, 1972) the hypothesis was retested for vowels. We found that when a vowel is heavily stressed, some of the muscles which are important for its formation increase in activity. This formulation is still incomplete, however. Any vowel placement is made by many muscles. The vowels we tested were high front vowels. The muscle tested was the genioglossus, which will act to hump and front the tongue. Consequently, if it is more active when the vowel is stressed, the tongue will be fronted more. However, the muscles which open the jaw are also active for such vowels; if they become more active also under stress, they will counteract the effect of the genioglossus. There must be a redistribution of energy among the muscles for each different stress allophone; consequently, Lindblom's explanation of a single target representation cannot be correct.

Coarticulation refers to the tendency of the articulators to assume a different position for a particular phone, depending on what phones precede and follow it – a phenomenon that is very common in speech. Indeed, Liberman (1970) suggests that the tendency of the vocal tract to be involved with several phones concurrently, at any given instant, is a basis for the failure to find invariant acoustic signals for them and also for the requirement that a listener be able to decode the speech wave, not merely to identify successive discrete segments. Anticipatory coarticulation – that is, the effect of the coming phone on the present one – is most often described, though both right-to-left and left-to-right effects can occur.

A study of MacNeilage and deClerk (1969), has shown that coarticulatory effects, are virtually omnipresent – that is, that the signals for a given phone are regularly affected both by the phone preceding it and by the phone following it, though effects extending over strings of more than two phones were not observed in this study. One effect seen in the study by MacNeilage and deClerk, and in more detail in a later study (Harris, 1971), is particularly troublesome for a theory of speech production that attempts to account for anticipatory coarticulation. It would be relatively easy to explain the phenomenon if it were a matter of simple time-smear of some aspects or features of the production of one phone into the time domain of another. However, these studies give some indication that different muscles are used to produce a given consonant when it precedes different vowels. Such findings, if solidly confirmed, would leave little hope of salvaging the concept that phoneme strings are realized on a unit-by-unit basis, with simple mechanical adjustments of timing.

Further studies are needed to determine the number of phones over which coarticulation occurs and what determines the length of the sequence. Essentially three types of models have been proposed. One hypothesis implicit in speech synthesis formulations (Mattingly, 1968; Kelly and Gerstman, 1961; Ohman, 1967b) is that each phone has an influence field of fixed size and that articulatory position at any moment in time is determined by the relative weights of the fields. A second point of view is that coarticulatory fields are determined by syllabic organization (Kozhevnikov and Chistovich, 1965). A third point of view (Henke, 1967) is that coarticulatory fields of a given phone vary with its feature components and their compatibility. Recent empirical work by Daniloff and Moll (1968) and by Amerman, Daniloff and Moll (1970) suggests that Henke's view is at least partly correct, but no general formulation of the details is presently available.

This account has taken, thus far, an older and fairly conventional view of what the segmental units of speech might be, i.e. phonemes as the abstract segmental units, allophones as their variant forms, and phones as the realized units. A different and probably more useful view is to consider speech in terms of features that occur in parallel and often extend over several segmental units. The phoneme can then be characterized as a bundle of distinctive features, a description that gained currency almost two decades ago (Jakobson, Fant and Halle, 1963). The recent works of Chomsky and Halle (1968), in particular, have given new prominence to feature-based descriptions. In their work, the string of phonemes has been replaced by a feature matrix as the phonetic representation that immediately precedes, and guides, a native speaker's production of the actual sounds. This matrix specifies the state of each feature of a phonetic segment.

Thus, the successive phonetic segments (each specified by its feature composition) correspond — though only approximately — to the string of extrinsic allophones in the older description.

The feature-matrix representation, since it is derived by successive transformations from an abstract, high-level form of the message rather than being inferred from speech itself, could hardly be expected to mesh perfectly with experimental observation. Thus, objections have been made, on phonetic and physiological grounds, to the particular feature systems which have been advanced by Chomsky, Halle and their co-workers.

An approach based on a feature description could, however, have important advantages, although it will almost surely be necessary to find features that are compatible with a dynamic physiological account of speech as well as with a linguistic description. A feature description is acceptable from a perceptual point of view, since features have perceptual reality — that is, listeners respond to place and manner cues independently, as shown by a wide variety of experimental studies. Dichotic listening tests, as in the recent study by Studdert-Kennedy and Shankweiler (1970), are particularly revealing. Another advantage of a feature description is that it provides flexibility in dealing with the time dimension in speech (Lisker, 1970). Thus, it eliminates such problems as the one mentioned above in connection with Ohman's numerical coarticulation model, namely, that all the effects of coarticulation were presumed to take place simultaneously for a given phoneme. Fant (1962) has discussed the segmentation of a short speech signal and has shown that most of its component acoustic segments include features that are associated with more than one phonetic segment, and that the time courses for the component features of a segment are not identical.

Another advantage of a feature description is that it allows the problem of coarticulation to be reformulated: instead of complex interactions between elusive segmental units, one deals with the temporal coordination of slowly changing, and essentially independent, features. Such a description would, indeed, be simple if the features derived from a linguistic description were to map directly onto the activities of distinct and independent parts of the articulatory apparatus, e.g. the several muscle systems that cause the articulators to move. But surely this is an oversimplification. The parts of the articulatory system are not truly independent and so the whole apparatus must have its actions coordinated, even if some of the activity is irrelevant for the speech signal; further, this kind of coordination may extend to preplanning that is aimed at the attainment of specific target shapes or sequences of target shapes of about syllabic size. Even so, the question of how the speech gestures are organized is transformed, by adopting a feature point of view, into one about physiologically-plausible events such as the timing of commands to the muscles and the complicating effects of mechanical linkages.

However, whether we deal with features or phonemes as the ultimate units of speech analysis, the failure to attain constant articulatory targets is not yet generally understood. One further question is how even approximate target maintenance is achieved. The usual explanation, as proposed by MacNeilage (1970) for example, is that this is done by feedback of some sort.

The assumption is that either tactile or kinesthetic information from the articulators is fed back in some form to the system that generates speech, i.e. that speech is, at least partially, under closed-loop control. Evidence that is usually offered in support of this position includes case studies of persons with gross somesthetic deficits where there is some evidence of accompanying gross defects in motor speech performance (MacNeilage, Rootes and Chase, 1967) instances of children with functional speech defects who can be shown to have impaired performance in oral stereognosis (Ringel *et al.,* 1970), and a long series of experiments beginning with the classic studies of Ringel and Steer (1963), that employ partial blockage of sensory feedback from the tongue and find impaired articulation. More recent examinations of the problem by Scott (1970), Butt (1970), Gammon, Smith, Daniloff and Kim (1971) and Borden (1972) have suggested that the impairment is rather small and is confined to a restricted class of articulatory events. Furthermore, it is unclear what neural functions are being eliminated by the nerve block procedure (see Scott for a discussion of this problem). A further complication is that a preliminary study by Borden (1972) suggests that some

presumed sensory effects of nerve block may be due to motor
paralysis of some of the extrinsic tongue muscles, as an artifact of
the procedure.

THE PHYSIOLOGICAL SUBSTRATE OF
SUPRASEGMENTAL AND MANNER GESTURES

Issues raised about the organization of speech are as pertinent
to a discussion of manner distinctions as they are to place
distinctions, but it will still be convenient to discuss these issues in
connection with voicing, oralization and intonation separately.

Laryngeal Organization for Pitch Control

The five intrinsic laryngeal muscles are traditionally divided into
three groups — tensors, abductors and adductors. The posterior
crico-arytenoid has normally been thought of as the sole abductor,
the crico-thyroid as a tensor, while the thyro-arytenoid is
sometimes considered to be a tensor and sometimes an adductor.
The lateral crico-arytenoids and inter-arytenoids are usually
designated as adductors (Sawashima, 1970).

Recent studies have concentrated on the regulation of pitch and
intensity. Four possible mechanisms have been suggested for pitch
control in running speech. First, pitch rises and falls are clearly
controlled by the activity of the tensors, the crico-thyroid and the
vocalis. This fact has been reconfirmed in several studies
(Faaborg-Andersen, 1957; Hirano, Ohala and Vennard, 1969; Gay,
Hirose, Strome and Sawashima, 1971) whether the pitch changes
are in singing or in running speech. A second possible mechanism
for changing pitch is by the action of the strap muscles of the
neck. This action is discussed below.

A third possible mechanism is by the action of subglottal
pressure on laryngeal vibration. This effect has been known for
some time (van den Berg, 1960). However, there has been
considerable controversy about its magnitude. Lieberman (1967)
has argued that the terminal pitch fall at the end of ordinary
declarative sentences is a result of the effect of fall in subglottal
pressure on the pitch contour. Ohala (1970) does not believe that

the subglottal pressure effect is substantial enough to account for the observed fall. He believes that it is caused by the strap muscles acting to lower pitch. Recent figures (Netsell, 1969) on subglottal pressure on pitch give a value for the effect which is intermediate between Lieberman's figure and Ohala's. However, further experimental work is necessary on possible interactions between increased subglottal pressure and laryngeal adjustment as a response.

One study (Gay, Hirose, Strome and Sawashima, 1971) shows that if a subject is asked to phonate with increased loudness, (and presumably, increased subvocal pressure, although this was not measured) the activity of intrinsic laryngeals does not increase very much, or very consistently, from subject to subject. However, further work on this point is clearly necessary.

A fourth possible mechanism should probably be mentioned for completeness. Different configurations of the upper vocal tract will have a back-loading effect on the frequency of laryngeal vibration (Flanagan and Landgraf, 1968). In other words, for any given subglottal pressure and laryngeal adjustment, there may be differences in fundamental frequency, depending on the shape of the upper vocal tract. Again, the magnitude of this effect is in question at the present time; it may well not be important in running speech.

The Action of the Strap Muscles of the Neck

There are three strap muscles of the neck — the sterno-thyroid, the thyro-hyoid and the sterno-hyoid. Their function in speech is somewhat obscure. Examination of their origins and insertions suggests that they can operate to open the jaw or to move the larynx. It is not clear whether their potential larynx moving action has direct effects on pitch. An earlier report (Sonninen, 1968) has shown that if the strap muscles are cut as part of a procedure for thyroidectomy, trained singers will lose the top note or two of their ranges. However, this result is not conclusive, since muscle use in trained singing may well not be like muscle use in speech. Ohala (1970) has shown that activity in the sterno-hyoid seems to be greater at the end of sentences, when the pitch falls. This result has not been confirmed by Garding, Fujimura and Hirose (1970). The Ohala result is complicated by the fact that the sterno-hyoid can be shown to open the jaw (Ohala and Hirose, 1970; Harris, 1971); jaw opening may have been a factor in Ohala's finding.

The sterno-thyroid has been found in preliminary results (Simada and Hirose, 1971) to be correlated with pitch falls in Japanese accent patterns. Again, its action can be shown to be correlated with jaw opening. Obviously, the whole question of the role of the strap muscles, and the more general problem of the role of external frame function in modifying intrinsic laryngeal adjustment, is in need of further investigation.

Laryngeal Action in Control of Segmental Gestures

The larynx serves as the primary sound source for speech. It operates in two modes — where the folds are retracted, a noise source results; when the cords are adducted, subglottal air drives them into vibration. In many languages of the world, voicing contrasts can be shown to be correlated with differences in the timing of a characteristic supraglottal occlusion and the abduction and adduction of the folds. This effect has been observed both indirectly, by examination of spectrograms (Lisker and Abramson, 1964) and directly, by viewing the larynx by the use of a fiberoptics system (Sawashima, Abramson, Cooper and Lisker, 1971).

More recently, it has been possible to assess the role of the various intrinsic laryngeal muscles in causing the opening and closing of the glottis in English stops (Hirose, 1971). Abduction of the folds is accomplished by the action of the posterior crico-arytenoid, and adduction by the action of the inter-arytenoids. These actions are in accord with traditional descriptions of the action of these muscles. However, Hirose's measurements show that the other two traditional adductors of the cords, the lateral crico-arytenoid and the thyro-arytenoid, do not seem to partici-pate in this opening and closing movement of the cords — that is, that there is functional differentiation among the so-called adductor muscles.

Lisker and Abramson (1971) believe that distinctions among

the stops are essentially conveyed by the changes in timing described above, and that accompanying changes are secondary. A more elaborate theory has been advanced by Chomsky and Halle (1968) and by Halle and Stevens (1971). In their view, voicing contrasts are the result of a complex set of orthogonal adjustments of subglottal systems, the larynx and the upper vocal tract. The apparent purpose of this scheme is to preserve the notion of a set of relatively steady state adjustments which will have consequences for laryngeal timing, but are not temporal in essence.

The crucial question for the study of the segmental voicing gesture is whether *voicing* distinctions can be considered a matter of laryngeal timing perhaps with correlated extra laryngeal maneuvers, or whether voicing can be fitted into a steady state schema of phonetic description. Further research is clearly necessary on this point. The one study we have made involves the pharyngeal adjustments concomitant with voicing. This study will be discussed in the section below.

The Physiology of the Oralization-Nasalization Dimension

Six muscles surround the velopharyngeal port. Due to the importance of velopharyngeal closure for intelligible speech and the commonness of the cleft palate problem, the velopharyngeal mechanism has perhaps seen more extensive physiological study than any other part of the oral area. The interested reader will find an extremely complete review of the literature in a monograph by Fritzell (1969).

The port is closed by the action of lifting the velum, primarily by the action of its largest muscle, the levator palatini; the secondary velar muscle, the tensor veli palatini, does not seem to function in speech (Fritzell, 1969).

The muscles which form the sides of the pharyngeal cavity seem to aid velar action by tensing for oral gestures and relaxing for nasal gestures (Lubker, Fritzell, and Lindquist, 1971; Berti and Hirose, 1972). These authors are in disagreement, however, over the function of the palatoglossus. Its anatomical location is such that it may have either of two opposing functions — it may aid in oralization by assisting the palatopharyngeus, or it may actively nasalize by pulling down on the velum. The two groups differ on which function it has in speech. The disagreement should be easily resolved by future research.

Pharyngeal Organization for Voicing

As we said above, it has been proposed by Chomsky and Halle that the control of voicing is not simply a matter of timing of the action of the laryngeal muscles, but involves a series of orthogonal adjustments of the upper vocal tract which will inhibit or promote vibration of the vocal folds. In particular, it has been proposed that the pharyngeal walls become tense to inhibit voicing, for the voiceless stops and lax to promote voicing, for the voiced. Kent and Moll (1969) have argued that pharyngeal enlargement may well be under active control. In a study of several of the muscles of the pharyngeal area, Berti (1971b) has shown that muscle activity may increase or decrease for a voiced sound, depending on whether the muscle will, by being active, increase or decrese pharyngeal area. Thus, the levator palatini, which increases vertical pharynx size, tends to be more active for voiced consonants, while the superior constrictor, which will decrease front-to-back diameter, is more active for voiceless sounds.

A further interesting aspect of this work is that, while all subjects studied will use some form of pharyngeal enlargement for voicing, they differ in which mechanism they choose. The effect of any enlargement is simply to increase the reservoir size for maintaining a transglottal pressure differential; there is no evidence that these mechanisms operate separately from glottal adjustment at this time.

THE FUTURE OF PHYSIOLOGICAL SPEECH RESEARCH

This chapter has attempted to summarize what we know now about some aspects of the coordination of articulation in speech. It is clear that at a purely descriptive level, some selected parts of the mechanism are quite well understood. However, at the level of understanding the organization of speech as the listener operates upon it, we have not advanced very much since the time of Daniel

Jones. Future research must lay heavy emphasis on attempts to understand the way that parts of the mechanism are coordinated, both in space and in time. There seems to be good reason to suppose that the techniques which have been so helpful in mapping should also prove useful in this more fundamental task.

REFERENCES

Amerman, J. D., Daniloff, R., and Moll, K. L.: Lip and jaw coarticulation for the phoneme /æ /. J Speech Hear Res, 13:147-161, 1970.

Berti, F. B.: The velopharyngeal mechanism: An electromyographic study — A preliminary report. Haskins Laboratories SR-25/26, 117-130, 1971.

Berti, F. B., and Hirose, H.: Velopharyngeal function in oral-nasal articulation and voicing gestures. Haskins Laboratories SR-28, 1972.

Borden, G. J.: Some effects of oral anesthesia on speech: a perceptual and electromyographic analysis. Ph.D. dissertation, City University of New York, 1972.

Butt, A. H.: The effects on speech of labial anesthesia: a photographic study. M.S. thesis, Purdue University, 1971.

Bzoch, K. R.: Assessment: radiographic techniques. ASHA Reports Number 5, 271-282, 1970.

Chomsky, N., and Halle, M.: The Sound Pattern of English. New York; Harper & Row, 1968.

Daniloff, R. G., and Moll, K. L.: Coarticulation of lip-rounding. J Speech Hear Res, 11:707-721, 1968.

Faaborg-Andersen, K.: Electromyographic investigation of intrinsic laryngeal muscles in humans. Acta Physiol Scand 41, Suppl. 140, 1957.

Fant, C. G. M.: Acoustic Theory of Speech Production. The Hague, Mouton, 1960.

Fant, C. G. M.: Descriptive analysis of the acoustic aspects of speech. Logos, 5:3-17, 1962.

Flanagan, J. L., and Landgraf, L. L.: Self-oscillating source for vocal tract synthesizers. IEEE Transactions on Audio & Electroacoustics, 16:57-64, 1968.

Fritzell, B.: The velopharyngeal muscles in speech. Acta Otolaryngol Suppl., 250, 1969.

Fromkin, V. A.: Neuromuscular specification of linguistic units. Lang Speech, 9:170-199, 1966.

Fromkin, V.: The non-anomolous nature of anomolous utterances. Language, 47:27-51, 1971.

Fujisaki, H., and Nakamura, N.: Normalization and recognition of vowels. Annual Report of the engineering Research Institute, Tokyo University, 28:61-66, 1969.

Gammon, S. A., Smith, P. J., Daniloff, R. G., and Kim, C. W.: Articulation and stress/juncture production under oral anesthetization and masking. J Speech Hear Res, 14:271-282, 1971.

Garding, E., Fujimura, O., and Hirose, H.: Laryngeal control of Swedish word tone — a preliminary report on an EMG study. Ann. Bulletin Research Institute of Logopedics and Phoniatrics, Tokyo University, No. 4:45-54, 1970.

Gay, T., and Harris, K. S.: Some recent developments in the use of electromyography in speech research. J Speech Hear Res, 14:241-246, 1971.

Gay, T., Hirose, H., Strome, M., and Sawashima, M.: Electromyography of the intrinsic laryngeal muscles during phonation. Haskins Laboratories SR-25/26, 97-106, 1971.

Halle, M., and Stevens, K.: A note on laryngeal features. MIT Research Laboratory of Electronics QPR 101, 198-211, 1971.   ·

Harris, K. S., Lysaught, G. F., and Schvey, M. M.: Some aspects of the production of oral and nasal labial stops. Lang Speech, 8:135-147, 1965.

Harris, K. S., Gay, T., Sholes, G. N., and Lieberman, P.: Some stress effects on electromyographic measures of consonant articulations. Proceedings of the 6th International Congress on Acoustics, Kyoto, Japan and Haskins Laboratories SR-13/14, 137-152, 1968.

Harris, K. S.: Physiological measures of speech movements: EMG and fiberoptic studies. ASHA Reports Number 5, 271-282, 1970.

Harris, K. S.: Action of the extrinsic musculature in the control of tongue position. Haskins Laboratories SR-25/26, 87-96, 1971.

Harris, K. S.: Vowel stress and articulatory reorganization. Haskins Laboratories SR-28, 1972.

Henke, W.: Preliminaries to speech synthesis based on an articulatory model. Conference Preprints, 1967 Conference on Speech Communication and Processing. Bedford, Air Force Cambridge Research Laboratories, 1967, pp. 170-177.

Hirano, M., and Ohala, J.: Use of hooked-wire electrodes for electromyography of the intrinsic laryngeal muscles. J Speech Hear Res, 12:362-373, 1969.

Hirano, M., Ohala, J., and Vennard, W.: The function of laryngeal muscles in regulating fundamental frequency and intensity of phonation. J Speech Hear Res., 12:616-628, 1969.

Hirose, H.: An electromyographic study of laryngeal adjustments during speech articulation: a preliminary report. Haskins Laboratories SR-25/26, 107-116, 1971.

Houde, R. A.: A study of tongue body motion during selected speech sounds. SCRL Monogr. No. 2, Santa Barbara: Speech Communications Research Laboratory, 1967.

Jakobson, R., Fant, C. G. M., and Halle, M.: Preliminaries to speech analysis. Cambridge, MIT Press, 1963. Originally published as Technical Report

No. 13, Acoustics Laboratory, M.I.T., 1963.

Kelly, J. L., and Gerstman, L.: An artificial talker driven by a phonetic input. J Acoust Soc Am, 33:835(A), 1961.

Kent, R. D., and Moll, K. L.: Vocal-tract characteristics of the stop cognates. J Acoust Soc Am, 46:1549-1555, 1969.

Kozhevnikov, V. A., and Chistovich, L. A.: Rech' Artikulyatsiya i Vospriyatiye, 1965. Translated as Speech: Articulation and Perception. Washington, Joint Publications Research Service, 30, 543, 1966.

Ladefoged, P., deClerk, J. L., and Harshman, R.: Factor analyses of tongue shapes. J Acoust Soc Am, 50:140(A), 1971.

Liberman, A. M.: The grammars of speech and language. Cognitive Psychology, 1:301-323, 1970.

Lieberman, P.: Intonation, perception and language. Cambridge, MIT Press, 1967.

Lindblom, B. E. F.: Spectrographic study of vowel reduction. J Acoust Soc Am, 35:1773-1781, 1963.

Lindblom, B. E. F., and Sundberg, J. E. F.: Acoustical consequences of lip, tongue, jaw, and larynx movement. J Acoust Soc Am, 50:1166-1179, 1971.

Lisker, L.: On time and timing in speech. Haskins Laboratories SR-23, 151-178, 1970.

Lisker, L., and Abramson, A. S.: A cross-language study of voicing in initial stops: acoustical measurements. Word, 20:384-422, 1964.

Lisker, L., and Abramson, A. S.: Distinctive features and laryngeal control. Language, 47:767-785, 1971.

Lubker, J. F.: An Electromyographic-cineradiographic investigation of velar function during normal speech production. Cleft Palate J, 5:1-18, 1968.

Lubker, J. F.: Aerodynamic and ultrasonic assessment techniques in speech-dentofacial research. ASHA Reports Number 5, 207-223, 1970.

Lubker, J. F., Fritzell, B., and Lindquist, J.: Velopharyngeal function: An electromyographic study. Royal Institute of Technology, STL-QPSR, 4:9-20, 1970.

MacNeilage, P. F., and Sholes, G. N.: An electromyographic study of the tongue during vowel production. J Speech Hear Res, 7:209-232, 1964.

MacNeilage, P. F., Rootes, T. P., and Chase, R. A.: Speech production and perception in a patient with severe impairment of somesthetic perception and motor control. J Speech Hear Res, 10:449-467, 1967.

MacNeilage, P. F., and deClerk, J. L.: On the motor control of coarticulation in CVC monosyllables. J Acoust Soc Am, 45:1217-1233, 1969.

MacNeilage, P. F.: Motor control of serial ordering of speech. Psychol Rev, 77:182-195, 1970.

Mattingly, I. G.: Synthesis by rule of general American English. Supplement to Haskins Laboratories SR, 1968.

Moller E.: The Chewing apparatus: an electromyographic study of the action of the muscles of mastication and its correlation to facial morphology.

Acta Physiol Scand, 69, Suppl. 280, 1966.

Netsell, R.: A perceptual-acoustic-physiological study of stress. Ph.D. dissertation, University of Iowa, 1969.

Ohala, J.: Aspects of the control and production of speech. Working Papers in Phonetics, UCLA, 15, 1970.

Ohala, J., and Hirose, H.: The function of the sternohyoid muscle in speech. Annual Bulletin Research Institute of Logopedics and Phoniatrics, Tokyo University, No. 4:41-44, 1970.

Öhman, S. E. G., Leandersson, R., And Persson, A.: EMG studies of facial muscle activity in speech. II. Royal Institute of Technology, STL-QPSR 1:1-4, 1966.

Öhman, S. E. G.: Numerical model of coarticulation. J Acoust Soc Am, 41:310-320, 1967b.

Öhman, S. E. G.: Peripheral motor commands in labial articulation. Royal Institute of Technology, STL-QPSR, 4:30-63, 1967a.

Perkell, J. S.: Physiology of Speech Production: Results and Implications of a Quantitative Cineradiographic Study. Cambridge, MIT Press, 1969.

Raphael, L. J.: An electromyographic investigation of the tense-lax feature in some English vowels. Haskins Laboratories SR-25/26:131-140, 1971.

Ringel, R. L., and Steer, M. D.: Some effects of tactile and auditory alterations on speech output. J Speech Hear Res, 6:369-378, 1963.

Ringel, R. L., House, A. S., Burk, K. W., Dolinsky, J. P., and Scott, C. M.: Some relations between orosensory discrimination and articulatory aspects of speech production. J. Speech Hear Disord 35:3-11, 1970.

Sawashima, M.: Laryngeal research in experimental phonetics. Haskins Laboratories SR-23, 69-116, 1970.

Sawashima, M., Abramson, A. S., Cooper, F. S., and Lisker, L.: Observing laryngeal adjustments during running speech by use of a fiberoptics system. Phonetica, 22:193-201, 1970.

Scott, C. M.: A phonetic analysis of the effects of oral sensory deprivation. Ph.D. dissertation, Purdue University, 1970.

Simada, Z., and Hirose, H.: Physiological correlates of Japanese accent patterns. Ann. Bulletin of Research Institute of Logopedics and Phoniatrics, Tokyo University No. 5:41-50, 1971.

Smith, T. J.: A phonetic study of the function of the extrinsic tongue muscles. Ph.D. dissertation, University California at Los Angeles, 1970.

Sonninen, A.: The external frame function in the control of pitch in the human voice. In Arendt Bouhuys (Ed.): Sound production in man, Annals of the New York Academy of Sciences, 155:68-89, 1968.

Stevens, K. N., and House, A. S.: An acoustical theory of vowel production and some of its implications. J Speech Hear Res, 4:303-320, 1961.

Studdert-Kennedy, M., and Shankweiler, D.: Hemispheric specialization for speech perception. J Acoust Soc Am, 48:579-594, 1970.

van den Berg, J.: Vocal ligaments versus registers. Current Problems in Phoniatrics and Logopedics, 1:19-34, 1960.

Van Riper, C., and Irwin, J. V.: Voice and Articulation. Englewood Cliffs, Prentice-Hall, 1958.

CHAPTER II

ORAL SENSATION AND PERCEPTION

ROBERT L. RINGEL

IT may be useful to view the speech production system as composed of control, effector and sensor units (Fairbanks 1954). In brief, it may be stated that the control unit stores and integrates sensory information and motor commands that are requisite for normal speech movements. The precise anatomic location of the control unit is not presently defined although it appears safe to assume that it is a cerebral mechanism. The function of the effector unit is to produce the motor actions necessary for speech production. The effector unit may be broken down for purposes of discussion into the sound source (respiratory mechanism), sound generator (larynx) and sound modulators (supra-glottic articulators). It is clear that failures in the function of the control and effector units result in articulation, voice and language disorders. A concept that may prove helpful when thinking about the action of the control and effector units of the speech production system is that they probably do not act independently of sensory information about their performance. Such information is often termed "feedback" and, according to some theorists, is essential for the development and maintenance of normal speech patterns. In fact, Hardy (1970) maintains that "while sensory and motor systems may be identified anatomically, their interaction is so necessary for appropriate muscular patterning that physiologically they must be considered in terms of the

NOTE: This chapter, with the exception of the introduction, has appeared previously under the title "Oral Sensation and Perception: A Selective Review" in *Speech and the Dentofacial Complex: The State of the Art.* ASHA Reports # 5, 188-206, 1970. Reproduced by permission of the American Speech and Hearing Association.

'sensorimotor systems.' "

Evidence which is generally used to support hypotheses concerning the importance of sensory feedback systems in the speech network has been drawn primarily from observations of the congenitally hearing impaired. In these persons the well documented observations of failure to develop normal speech are attributed to the inability of the speaker to monitor his own speech efforts. Indeed, the *primary* sensor unit in the early Fairbanks model of the speech system is the *auditory* channel which feeds information to the controller unit for subsequent adjustment of effector units. Attention to the role of audition in the speech production system has resulted in the development of tests to assess hearing acuity, discrimination, retention and perhaps even more important, techniques for compensating for disorders of this sensory input channel.

Early theories which viewed the speech system as a servo-mechanism relegated the *somesthetic* afferent systems to a secondary role by indicating that although they may supply information about the *mechanical operation* of the speech mechanism, they may give little direct information about its output (Hardy, 1970). Since then, however, it has been shown — in persons with acquired deafness, as well as in normal hearing persons under the influence of delayed auditory feedback or auditory masking — that effective reduction of the auditory sensor operation exhibits a relatively minimal immediate effect on articulation. These findings suggest that other afferent (feedback) systems such as those associated with taction and proprioception are involved in speech production.

Until recently, relatively little attention has been given to the potential role of the tactile and proprioceptive feedback channels in the speech production system. In light of recent experimental findings which emphasize sensory and perceptual experiences as an important element in the development and regulation of speech activities, background information about afferent systems and their role in normal and disordered speech would appear to be of value to the speech pathologist. It is hoped that the information contained in this chapter will be useful to the speech pathologist in the formation of diagnostic and therapeutic constructs and to the speech scientist in the development of models of the speech production system.

Failures in oral sensory and perceptual experiences often indicate nervous system pathology. Recent interest in oral sensation and perception, however, goes beyond its diagnostic value. The role of sensory and perceptual experiences in developing and regulating oral motor performance is currently being studied. It is now apparent that the finely coordinated motions of the mouth do not result from an array of spatially and temporally patterned motor impulses released blindly into the efferent network from high centers in the nervous system. Motor patterns are modified and restructured along the control pathway at various motor relay regions in accordance with information received from peripheral sensory resources (Paillard, 1960). Various theories attempt to explain some aspects of oral motor control as a feedback-level mechanism. Representative of such orientations are those concerned with speech production. It is not my intent to endorse any particular theory of speech control or to present all aspects of controversies surrounding such theories, nor is it to be implied that proprioceptive feedback is always a major component of the theory.

Fairbanks (1954) presented one of the most widely cited models of speech production calling for sensory monitoring of motor activity. The essentials of this system are

> feedback of the output to the place of control, comparison of the output with the input and such manipulation of the output producing device as will cause the output to have the same functional form as the input. (p.135)

More recent concepts of speech production systems give sensory processes relatively little attention. MacNeilage (1970) notes that

> at no point in these models was the active use of information from ongoing movement accorded a role which affected their form in a critical way, even though the possible influence of such mechanisms was sometimes noted. In fact, one of the main properties of these models is that the command system is independent of the peripheral response apparatus. (p. 186)

One can argue that the more recent models have been designed to account primarily for the motor control of the serial ordering of speech; such constructs attempt to specify the nature of the motor units at higher-to-lower levels in the articulation process. Recently MacNeilage has recognized that it may be necessary as well as enlightening to specify certain sensory mechanisms which may be operating, in order to explain context-dependent articulatory phenomena.

The extent to which sensory feedback processes have been included in models of the speech system varies with the nature of the model. Henke (1967) suggests that proprioceptive feedback provides the mechanisms whereby the timing or rate of articulatory activities is accomplished. As an example of the use of this kind of feedback, Henke describes the production of a stop in which ongoing articulation waits until contact between articulators (closure) is attained and then uses awareness of this happening, presumably through proprioceptive feedback, as a trigger for further articulatory activity. This view, of course, is not supported by some recent coarticulation data which shows that articulatory gestures often do not depend on the execution of antecedent articulatory events.

MacNeilage (1970), discussing the sequencing of articulatory movements, refers to the results of oral stereognosis studies as evidence that persons

> can integrate complex patterns of tactile and motor information to make accurate judgments of the spatial characteristcs of the stimulus objects. (p. 188)

He reasons further that

> it is likely that by such integration of motor information with concurrent tactile and other somesthetic and kinesthetic information (and auditory information) the language learner builds up an internalized spatial representation of the oral area. Within this representation he is able to signify points which must be reached for the articulation of various speech sounds, and because of the constant association of motor activity with development of the representation, he is readily able to specify the motor actions necessary for an articulator to reach a given target point. (p. 188)

Perkell (1969) views the speech production mechanism as composed of "two neuromuscular systems with different behavioral characteristics responding in general to different feedback." In his view of the articulation system, vowels are produced through the action of a slow extrinsic tongue muscle network under the primary influence of acoustic and myotactic feedback. Consonant production, on the other hand, is thought of as being produced by the combined function of the fast-acting intrinsic, as well as the slower extrinsic, muscle systems and is regulated by intraoral air pressure and tactile feedback. Ladefoged (1967) has also hypothesized that the production of vowels depends more on auditory monitoring than do the consonants, which depend more on oral sensory feedback.

Ladefoged (1967) questions whether the perception, as well as control, of speech is related to proprioceptive feedback mechanisms. Liberman (1957) presented a model of phonological perception in which speech production and perception are considered as two aspects of the same process. This model, which has resulted in the formation of the "motor theory" of speech perception, maintains that the acoustic stimulus leads to a covert articulatory response, the proprioceptive feedback of which leads to the discriminative event we call perception. The rationale underlying this theory has been expressed by Liberman and his associates (1961) as follows:

> We believe that in the course of his long experiences with language a speaker (and listener) learns to connect speech sounds with their appropriate articulations. In time, these articulatory movements and their sensory feedback (or, more likely, the corresponding neurological processes) become part of the perceiving process, mediating between the acoustic stimulus and its ultimate perception. (p. 177)

If this theory is tenable, then relating a listener's perception of speech exclusively to the acoustic correlates of the auditory sensation overlooks a potentially important perceptual system, namely, a listener's proprioceptive (kinesthetic) feedback mechanism.* To Ladefoged (1967), sole attention to the acoustic stimuli and neglect of a listener's own experiences as a producer is

> rather like trying to discuss the visual identification of the shapes of tables and chairs exclusively in terms of the photic stimulation of the retina, and without recognizing that the observer might organize his perceptions in terms of objects with which he is familiar. (p. 162)

The acceptance of views about speech processes such as those described must be based on the demonstration of an oral sensory

---

*For a critical review of the motor theory of speech perception, see Lane (1965).

system in which the receptors are capable of providing the speaker with accurate information about his articulators and a neural system which is capable of relaying information received at the periphery to higher centers in the nervous system. In addition, support for the sensory component of the theoretically proposed systems of speech production should be available in evidence collected from the study of persons in whom the oral sensory system functions at different levels of proficiency.

In this chapter I will review evidence reflecting on the tenability of the speech system models. This information has been drawn primarily from neuroanatomic and physiologic studies as well as from investigations that have used the following research approaches: (1) tests of oral sensitivity; (2) detailed studies of persons with sensory pathologies and (3) experimentally induced sensory deficiencies. Finally, the chapter will highlight certain areas requiring additional research.

NEUROANATOMIC AND PHYSIOLOGIC STUDIES

Cutaneous Receptors

There are a wide variety of receptors throughout the oral mucosa. Grossman and Hattis (1967) summarized the distribution of these sensory endings and made some general statements about the neurohistologic makeup of the oral mucosa. They indicated that despite the diversity in size of sensory endings noted throughout the oral mucosa, and despite specific variations of innervation from site to site, there is a gross similarity in receptor form and in the pattern of innervation of the several oral surfaces. They also noted the declining progression of nerve-ending occurrence, generally from the front to the rear of the mouth, that is evident particularly in the tongue and hard palate, and that lingual sensory terminations are more numerous on the dorsal than on the inferior aspects. Grossman and Hattis commented that, in their view, low threshold to sensory experience exhibited by the mouth, when compared with that of skin surfaces, may be due to the presence of epithelial fibrillar extensions which are limited to moist mucous membranes.

With few exceptions, the presence in the oral mucosa of the receptor types and distributions described is accepted. The contribution of such information, however, toward understanding sensation and perception is still unresolved. According to Von Frey's classical concept, cutaneous sensations such as pain, cold, warmth and touch are subserved by specific receptors (Rose and Mountcastle, 1959). Research at Oxford University (Sinclair, 1955) which failed to relate specific endings to certain cutaneous modalities in several skin areas did not support the classic concept. The theory offered instead is known as the Pattern Theory and states that different cutaneous sensations arise not as a result of stimulation of a specific receptor type but rather because different stimuli affect the same receptor complex in a different manner.

As Rose and Mountcastle (1959) commented, however,

> one hesitates to accept as a solution to the vexing problem of the morphology of the encapsulated endings a declaration that virtually all morphological differences between them are either insignificant or due to artifacts of the technique. (p. 390)

More recently Melzack and Wall (1962) attempted to resolve the differences between the specific receptor and pattern theories by proposing that

> receptors are specialized physiologically for the transduction of particular kinds and ranges of stimuli into patterns of nerve impulses . . . and that every discriminable different somesthetic perception is produced by a unique pattern of nerve impulses. (p. 342)

This view has gained relatively widespread acceptance.

Muscle Receptors

It seems clear that information from cutaneous receptors reaches a cortical level via the trigeminal lemniscal system and that tactile information surely must contribute to conscious knowledge of articulatory position or kinesthesia. However, since running speech is certainly a highly automated motor act, it is appropriate to ask whether the oral structures contain receptors capable of contributing to reflex knowledge of articulator position or proprioception. Receptors such as those embedded in muscle spindles are known to have the capability to act in such a manner.

The muscle spindle is a specialized receptor unit in the muscle which contains polar intrafusal muscle fibers and central noncontractile sensory endings. The spindle intrafusal fibers are innervated by small-diameter gamma motoneurons and the spindle sensory neurons end in synaptic relations to the alpha motoneurons innervating the main body of the muscle. In this way a reflex arc is formed whereby a gamma motoneuron firing causes intrafusal fiber stretch on spindle sensory endings, which, in turn, fire and activate alpha motoneurons. Consequently, extrafusal fibers contract until spindle sensory stretch is eliminated. This functional mechanism has been referred to as the *gamma loop.*

Controversy exists both about the presence of muscle spindles in oral structures such as the tongue and about their possible importance in oral sensory functioning. While Blom (1960) found no such receptors in the tongue, Cooper (1953) observed muscle spindles in the region of the tongue proximal to the tip. Rose and Mountcastle (1959) cited two pieces of evidence which argue against the inclusion of muscle spindles as a kinesthetic sensing device. First, the discharge rate of muscle spindles has been shown to be unrelated to muscle length, whereas joint receptor discharge rate seems to relate to muscle tension. Second, spindle afferents seem to relay to the cerebellum but not to the postcentral cortex. Thus, information from muscle spindles is not available for conscious introspection in motor learning (Shelton, in press). Matthews (1964) reported that it is widely accepted that muscle spindles are not primarily important for any contribution they make to conscious awareness of position.

Investigators who attach some importance to muscle spindles in the control of speech production, however, generally have not believed that conscious perception of position is a necessary requisite. Rather, the muscle spindle is thought to be important not in the sense that it is like primary sensory receptors but because it is a structural component of the gamma efferent loop. MacNeilage (1970) postulated that the motor commands for invariant target positions (states of muscle contraction in the vocal tract) may be issued via gamma motoneurons.

He states:

As a gamma command of a given magnitude will always require the main body of the muscle to assume the same length in order to eliminate stretch on the sensory fibers, the gamma loop appears to be a mechanism whereby a muscle can attain the same position regardless of its length preceding the gamma command. (p. 191)

If the gamma loop is to function in the manner MacNeilage hypothesizes, an explanation of the inevitable *time loss* in neural transmission around the loop is necessary. Matthews (1964) discusses the gamma loop delay problem and draws an analogy between the gamma efferent system and inanimate servo-control systems in which time delays, and their resultant system oscillations, are counteracted by mechanisms within the loop which predict the nature of the *end* signal. With specific reference to the gamma loop, Matthews views the primary afferent muscle spindle endings as a potential compensatory mechanism for the time delay, since they are responsive to the velocity of muscle spindle stretch and capable of using such information about the rate of muscle change

to "predict" the length of the muscle after the delay time of the reflex, and so ensure that the response will be appropriate to the time when the reflex becomes effective, rather than to the earlier time when the reflex was initiated. (p. 278)

If this latter view is correct, the gamma loop mechanism may be an important component in oral sensory functioning for speech.

An example of the role that proprioceptive feedback might play in the control of speech activities is contained in the work of Kirchner and Wyke (1964, 1965). Their investigations have revealed that the larynx is equipped with two distinct intrinsic mechanoreceptor reflex systems, one a phasic reflex system which is driven from rapidly adapting receptors located in the capsules of the laryngeal joints (the articular system) and the other a tonic servoreflex system which is driven from slowly adapting receptors embedded within the muscles themselves (the myotatic system). These systems clearly play a part in the continuous and precise adjustment of laryngeal muscle tone during phonation.

In brief, Wyke (1967) has stated that, once the column of air is set into motion within the larynx, the laryngeal muscles and the cartilages to which they are attached are deflected from their preset phonatory posture:

It is the function of the articular and myotatic reflex systems within the larynx to return the muscles promptly to the desired coordinated pattern of contraction and relaxation, and to keep them there, during the period of phonatory air flow.

Finally, once the sound becomes audible, further adjustments are made (both voluntarily and reflexly) to the tone of the respiratory, laryngeal, buccopharyngeal and labio-glossal musculature in response to acoustic monitoring of the subject's own vocal performance. (p. 13)

The work of Kawamura (1965) on the mandibular musculature also supports the presence of a sensory control mechanism for motor activity. He reports:

A noxious stimulus to the oral and perioral structures will easily induce the jaw-opening reflex. There are close connections between the sensory nucleus of the trigeminal nerve and its motor nucleus which innervate the jaw muscles. Noxious stimuli to the oral structures have some inhibitory or facilitatory effects on the motor nucleus of the trigeminal nerve, and oral sensations may regulate the jaw muscles activities by means of this feedback system. (p. 182)

In Kawamura's view, motor control of the jaw muscles is primarily a function of sensory processes originating within the temporomandibular joint (TMJ). Specifically, he believes that information from the mandibular sensory systems is transmitted to the trigeminal nuclei and that close connections exist between the sensory nucleus of the trigeminal nerve, which receives the afferent signals, and its motor nucleus, which innervates the mandibular musculature. Kawamura (1961) has also reported that certain types of oral stimuli tend to inhibit or facilitate motor activities of the jaw. Thus it appears that the sensory experiences of the TMJ may regulate and otherwise control mandibular motor activity by means of a feedback system. More specifically, the sensory mechanisms of the TMJ are hypothesized to play an active role in regulating the tension and length of jaw muscles, the position of the mandible, the maintenance of the *free-way space* (oral aperture) and the dynamics of mandibular movements.

TESTS OF ORAL SENSITIVITY

There is a rapidly growing body of literature dealing with the oral sensory abilities of pathological groups of speakers. The underlying intent of such investigations has been to establish whether or not a measurable relationship exists between oral sensory functioning and speaking proficiency. The most common method of assessment has been that of oral form recognition. In a typical test of oral form recognition, a subject is asked to orally manipulate a previously unseen three-dimensional form and to identify that form from a group of visually presented forms. Tests developed by various investigators (the development of oral form-recognition tests has a short but extensive history which has been reviewed recently by Shelton, 1970) have differed in number and type of form used, as well as the exact nature of the task required of subjects. These methodological differences place certain limitations on the comparison of results that I shall describe and may account for some of the conflicting results and conclusions.

The speakers studied most extensively with tests of oral form recognition are those with articulation defects in the absence of known organic or structural pathologies. Four separate investigations (Moser *et al.*, 1967; Ringel, Burk and Scott, 1968; Ringel *et al.*, 1970; Weinberg, Lyons and Liss, 1970) have demonstrated that articulatory-defective speakers have more difficulty with oral form recognition than do their normal-speaking controls. This has been demonstrated for children as well as adults (Ringel *et al.*, 1970). In addition to the generally positive relation between articulation skill and oral form performance, it has been demonstrated that measurements of oral form discrimination can differentiate between degrees of articulatory proficiency that have been established a priori by independent means (Ringel, Burk and Scott, 1968). Thus, children and adults with mild articulatory problems make more errors than normals, but significantly fewer errors than speakers with more severe articulation problems. In an interesting investigation, Locke (1968) showed that children with good oral-form scores are better able to learn unique articulatory tasks than children with poor oral form skill (Moser, LaGourgue and Class, 1967; Arndt, Elbert and Shelton, 1970).

Oral form recognition also has been employed to assess sensory abilities in cerebral palsy, cleft palate and stuttering. In a group of athetoid patients, Solomon (1965) reported that form recognition was positively correlated with ratings of chewing and drinking ability and with articulation scores. In the Moser, LaGourgue and Class (1967) study, cerebral-palsied adults made oral form judgments which were significantly poorer than those of their normal controls. They also reported that a group of stutterers made poor oral form judgements in an investigation by Hochberg and Kabcenell (1967), while Mason (1967) found that normal and cleft-palate speakers behaved similarly.

A less-frequently employed tool for evaluating sensation in pathological speakers is two-point discrimination. Schliesser (1965) found two-point discrimination in the lip to be positively correlated with speech defectiveness in spastic hemiplegic children. Patients with muscular dystrophy and concurrent speech difficulties demonstrated larger limen and variability values than did normal subjects in a recent investigation (Ringel, 1970). On the other hand, Rutherford and McCall (1967) were unable to show significant two-point limen differences between normal and cerebral-palsied children, and Addis (1968) found that limen values for stutterers are like those of normal speakers.

Examples of the application of other methods of assessing oral sensation in pathologic groups can be found in the literature. These include methods designed to measure tactile acuity, texture discrimination, localization, pattern recognition, kinesthetic pattern recognition and vibrotactile sensitivity and scaling (Rutherford and McCall, 1967; Fucci, 1968). In general, these methodologies have not discriminated between pathologic and normal speakers as well as oral form testing procedures.

As noted, oral form-recognition testing most often has been employed in evaluating sensory capabilities in clinical groups of speech-defective individuals. It is probably true that the factor of clinical expediency explains, in part, the widespread use of oral form-recognition in assessing sensory abilities. In most of its forms, the test is relatively easy to administer and can be accommodated by fairly young children as well as by individuals with severely handicapping conditions such as cerebral palsy and muscular dystrophy. More interesting, however, is the attempt to explain why this task seems to relate to a skill such as speech.

Since many studies of oral form recognition have been concerned largely with methodological questions and factors such as test reliability, they have not asked this question. A notable exception is found in the writing of Shelton, Arndt and Hetherington (1967). These authors recognized the necessity of attempting to describe both anatomically and physiologically the nature of the task of oral form recognition and state, "the ability to recognize forms orally requires the integrity of both peripheral receptors for touch and kinesthesis and also central integrating processes." We (Ringel *et al.*, 1970) have also alluded to this problem in a statement about performance on an oral form-discrimination task:

> It is not enough to believe that the severity of an oral discrimination disability increases merely as the total error score increases; identification of the level of discrimination failure is crucial for understanding the sensory deficit in question and its potential effect on organized motor activities of speech production. (p. 4)

Variables which appear to affect oral sensory performance also have been investigated. For example, performance levels have been shown to improve with increasing age through midadolescence, when these levels seem to stabilize, as demonstrated by Arndt, Elbert and Shelton (1970). McDonald and Aungst (1967) obtained similar results for oral form recognition and demonstrated that mean scores decreased considerably in a geriatric population. We (Ringel *et al.*, 1970) reported that articulatory-defective adults performed better in oral form discrimination than did normal-speaking children with a mean age of eight years. These facts strongly suggest that age facilitates performance in oral form-discrimination. Maturational indices can be discussed as having at least two major components — one related to physiological abilities as such and the other involving *higher orders* or organization of input to the organism. The adult may be more proficient in stimulus exploration than the child because of superior motor abilities that permit more appropriate manipulation of the stimulus forms. Similarly, the increased ratio of oral-cavity size to stimulus-form size in the adult as compared to the child may favor more adequate manipulation. Other factors which may favor the adult in discriminating form include his more developed motivational attitudes and his attention and retention spans.

Testing of the oral region has shown that the oral cavity does not demonstrate uniformity in its mode of response to stimulation. Certain regions of the oral cavity are more capable of making perceptual evaluations than others, and different stimuli depend on different oral regions for their successful evaluation. In general, research in two-point discrimination indicates that the front of the mouth is more sensitive than its posterior regions and that increased discriminability exists at the midline of the structure (Ringel and Ewanowski, 1965). Grossman, Hattis and Ringel (1965) reported that the lip exhibited more sensitive tactile thresholds than the incisive papilla. However, the tongue is capable of more accurate texture judgments than the lips (Ringel and Fletcher, 1967). McCall and Kirkley (1967) demonstrated bilateral symmetry for tactile thresholds in the lower lip. Arndt, Elbert and Shelton (1970) observed that fewer forms were identified when explored by the lips alone than the entire oral cavity and tongue. This seems to indicate that oral form recognition is a skill for which lingual sensitivity and manipulation are paramount. Some recent research on the palate by Shelton *et al.* (in press) would seem to indicate that kinesthesia is poorer for movement of the palate than for other parts of the body.

In general, the results of studies which have tested various parameters of oral sensitivity indicate that the progression from maximal to minimal discrimination involves the lingual, labial and palatal structures, in that order, and that the lingual region rivals the fingertip in relative sensitivity. An evaluation of these findings has been reported (Ringel and Ewanowski, 1965). The reviewed literature indicated that

> the discriminatory ability of an area varies directly with the size of its cortical and thalamic projection areas . . . the relative volume of tissue of the thalamic relay nuclei and of the post-central cortical gyrus which is devoted to a given peripheral area is directly related to the density of peripheral neural innervation of that region and inversely related to the size of the receptive fields contained within this peripheral area. (p. 395)

The finding of greatest sensitivity for the relatively mobile oral structures is also compatible with the observation that a correspondence exists between the mobility of a structure and its discriminatory ability (Silverman, 1961; Shewchuk and Zubek, 1960).

STUDIES OF PERSONS WITH SENSORY PATHOLOGIES

Intensive study of individual cases can provide insight into the role of oral sensation and perception. Such an investigation of a young woman with a congenital sensory deficit has been reported. Data from medical and developmental history, results of physical and neurological examinations, as well as results of nonvocal motor testing and histological investigation, are presented in some detail by Chase (1967). Rootes and MacNeilage (1967) reported the results of tests of speech perception, electromyography of the oral area and phonetic analysis of the patient's speech. Finally, Bosma (1967) has presented palatographic and cineradiographic data. The integration of such extensive data, and somewhat less-detailed data for another youngster with a similar oral sensory deficit (Bosma, 1967), bring to light a number of observations of potential significance in understanding sensation as it relates to skilled motor acts such as speech. For example, these patients' speech was described as minimally intelligible with consonant production being severely impaired; yet both were able to perceive light touch throughout the oral area. Such observations indicate that looking at types of sensations other than those embodied in *light touch* is requisite to understand speech monitoring. In this respect it is interesting to note that these patients were almost totally unable to perform on tasks of oral form recognition which, as discussed earlier, is often viewed as a skill requiring fairly high-level sensory function.

In one of these patients, the relation between speech perception and production also was investigated (Rootes and MacNeilage, 1967). This study was prompted by interest in the motor theory of speech perception discussed earlier. The investigators reported

> evidence in this subject that production and perception are inter-related, namely in front vowels and voiced stop consonants, where the most efficiently produced phones (/i/ and /b/) are also the ones most successfully identified. (p. 317)

Rootes and MacNeilage urged caution in interpreting these results, however, since the patient's perception of speech in informal conversation was considerably better than would be predicted, in accordance with the motor theory, from her speech production alone. In another interesting case study, McDonald and Aungst (1970) comment on "the apparent independence of oral sensory functions and articulatory proficiency." In their study of a cerebral-palsied patient they found good oral sensory capacities but very poor speech patterns.

EXPERIMENTALLY INDUCED SENSORY DEFICIENCIES

Since 1960, a series of studies have attempted to delineate the role of sensory mechanisms in speech through the use of nerve-blocking techniques that are assumed to induce temporary peripheral sensory lesions in the oral cavity (McCroskey, 1958; McCroskey, Corley and Jackson, 1959; Weber, 1961; Ringel and Steer, 1963; Ladefoged, 1967; Schliesser and Coleman, 1968; Thompson, 1969; Gammon, Smith, Daniloff and Kim, 1971; Scott and Ringel, 1971 a and b). The need for tests of the assumptions underlying this research is discussed later in this chapter.

A careful comparison of these investigations reveals certain points of agreement as well as disagreement. All investigators agree that speech resulting from tactile-kinesthetic deprivation remains highly intelligible. In other words, listeners have little difficulty *understanding* the speech of sensory-deprived talkers. This seems to be true for both single words and connected speech material and applies also to those conditions in which sensory deprivation and auditory masking are combined. This finding is of particular interest in light of the observations reported earlier for the two patients with the sensory system pathology whose speech was minimally intelligible. Since the intelligibility of speech under anesthesia is minimally affected, while it is seriously degraded in persons with congenital oral sensory deficits, it may be profitable to distinguish between anesthetized persons who have had normal oral sensory experiences in the past and those patients who have never experienced normal sensation in the mouth; or, at a different level, between those patients with a central sensory deficit and those with a loss of peripheral sensation. It does appear that in the short-term sense, the speech-producing mechanism is capable of maintaining a high degree of integrity (as reflected in speech intelligibility) in the presence of an interruption in its usual sources of information. Failure to induce speech alterations through anesthetization of the type observed in persons with congenital sensory deficits is provacative "in view of the stress placed by current speech control theory upon the importance of auditory and tactile feedback" (Schliesser and Coleman, 1968).

Studies also agree that tactile-kinesthetic deprivation results in certain phonetically observable changes and that consonants generally are perceived as being more affected than vowels. While the observations about vowels have been made a number of times and generally are accepted, this finding should not be interpreted to mean that the anesthetization procedures affect articulators less during vowel production, but rather may be merely a reflection of the fact that there is a wider degree of articulatory latitude which is phonetically tolerable in vowels. Most studies looking closely at the types of articulatory errors have pointed to the relative vulnerability of stops and fricatives to sensory deprivation. Similarly, the performances of subjects on certain non-speech tasks indicate that diadochokinetic rates are not affected by oral anesthetization but that performance on oral form-recognition tasks deteriorate under such conditions (Schliesser and Coleman, 1968; Gammon, Smith, Daniloff and Kim, 1971).

A major area of disagreement exists in the specific description of articulatory changes under anesthesia. McCroskey (1959) reported that most articulatory changes were of the substitution type. Gammon *et al.* (1971) concur with McCroskey and state that "the majority of mistakes occur as a result of changes from one manner or place to another rather than within such classes." On the other hand, three investigations have shown that articulatory changes are largely distortions. Ringel and Steer (1963) reported that listeners described most errors as distortions. Ladefoged (1967) stated that "one consonant was seldom replaced by another different enough to change the meaning, although this is a very common type of speech defect." Finally, in unpublished work now in preparation at Purdue University (Cheryl Scott and Ringel), it is observed that the overwhelming majority of articulatory changes under anesthesia were of the distortion type.

Whereas most studies noted previously used nerve-blocking procedure to achieve states of oral-region sensory deprivation, literature also exists on studies which used topical anesthetization techniques (Ringel and Steer, 1963; Henja, 1962; Ladefoged, 1967; Weiss, 1969). In general, these studies have reported that topical anesthetization has a minimal effect on speech accuracy. The one notable exception to this consensus is found in the work of Ladefoged (1967), who reported "very disorganized" although intelligible speech under topical anesthesia conditions. If the assumption is plausible that *light touch* is somewhat akin to the type of sensation that is disturbed in topical anesthetization and the case histories reported earlier are recalled, in which the patients' speech was poor but light touch sensation relatively normal, the role of light touch in speech monitoring must be questioned.

Perhaps the most interesting aspect of sensory deprivation investigations is the explanations of the data. McCroskey, Corley and Jackson (1959), like most of the later researchers, observed that semivowel and nasal-consonant production was relatively unaffected by tactile-kinesthetic deprivation. They reasoned that since semivowels and nasal-continuants are distinguished from other consonants mainly because of a durational difference (that is, they are longer), there exists a critical duration where monitoring responsibilities are shifted from tactile to auditory channels. This reasoning seems untenable, since it is not clear that fricatives, the class of consonants probably most affected by deprivation, are *short* sounds.

In earlier work (Ringel, 1962) no attempt was made to explain the specific effects of tactile-kinesthetic deprivation by itself. Rather, speech trends were explained in terms of general sensory alteration, both tactile-kinesthetic and auditory. Theoretical explanations were based on the hypothesized existence and accuracy of Fairbanks' servosystem theory of speech control. Articulatory inaccuracy was hypothesized to result from the comparator's inability, in the absence of sensory information, to perform its matching operation. Unable to compare actual output with intended output, the system is thus incapable of resolving errors. Decreased rate and increased amplitude of speech were attributed to the system's attempt to restore homeostasis to the speech process. Thus, the speaker slows down in an effort to increase the available time in which he might learn something about his speech. He speaks more loudly in an effort to compensate for disorganized information by increasing the total amount of information.

Ladefoged (1967) accounted for the differences in the effects of tactile versus auditory deprivation by ascribing distinctive functions to both channels. Vowel quality, nasality and pitch typically are monitored by reference to their acoustic properties, while consonant production is monitored through the oral sensory channel. Gammon, Daniloff and Smith (1971) have looked to the underlying articulatory differences between consonants in their attempts to explain the differential effects of sensory deprivation. The tendency for intended fricatives to become stops was expected, since the stop open-close articulation requires much less articulator precision and feedback than the precise constriction requirements for fricatives. These authors also reasoned that vowel production is monitored by kinesthetic feedback (rather than tactile feedback), which they did not consider to be disrupted by the nerve-block procedure. Similarly, stress/juncture production was hypothesized to depend on kinesthetic feedback.

The tendency to assign monitoring responsibilities for different types of articulatory events (for example, vowels and consonants) to separate sensory channels is premature in light of available evidence. Before accepting such a notion, considerable physiologic evidence on the nature of articulatory changes under conditions of deprivation is needed. In the production of a stop, for example, we need to know whether a speaker uses tactile information about a closure, as Henke (1967) hypothesizes, or if he relies more on some sense of intraoral pressure feedback. It is also important that the experimental data be consistent with clinical observations of the speech of the adventitiously deafened. To illustrate this latter point, Ladefoged's (1967) observation that consonants depend on tactile feedback would not explain the numerous consonant misarticulations characteristic of the deaf.

Two general statements can be made about the early tactile-kinesthetic deprivation studies. First, the investigations were, in effect, merely demonstrations of the often hypothesized relationship between tactile-kinesthetic sensation and speech production. That is, early tactile-kinesthetic deprivation studies demonstrated that speech changes result from oral sensory alteration. Secondly, as noted in the explanations of the differential effects of deprivation, the tendency was to assign monitoring responsibilities for unaffected articulatory events to other sensory channels presumed undisturbed by the anesthesia (auditory or kinesthetic). This reasoning reflects the belief that all types of articulatory activities are monitored by some sensory channel and is also another indication of the general acceptance of the speech servosystem theory.

It is conceivable, however, that other explanations may be needed to explain the differential effects of sensory deprivation on speech. Contrary to the views expressed in the Fairbanks model, it is possible that some motor commands received by the articulatory apparatus are not altered by the nature of tactile-kinesthetic information. Scott and Ringel have noted the importance of this issue and have hypothesized that a closed-loop tactile-kinesthetic feedback system may not operate for all types of articulatory activities. The presence of *open loop* control for certain articulatory activities along with *closed loop* control of other articulatory movements has also been theorized by MacNeilage (in press). The observation presented previously with regard to the case studies would seem to support this view. That is, tactile information about articulatory contacts made during the production of some consonants may not contribute crucial data to the feedback mechanism operating for speech. Finally, theories concerning the dominance of one type of feedback over another might be expanded to include considerations of *critical age* and type of feedback relationships. For example, it is quite plausible that the type of feedback important during a speech acquisition stage of development is different from that type which controls already acquired and stabilized speech activities. Failures to account for this view may help explain the poor correlations that are often reported between sensory skill capacities and speech proficiency. In other words, an adult's failure or excellence of performance on a sensory task does not yield much insight into the sensory level at which the subject functioned during an earlier, and perhaps even more critical, time.

FUTURE RESEARCH DIRECTIONS

Perhaps the most basic and critical question that remains to be resolved deals with the exact nature and relative importance of tactile and kinesthetic feedback in the development and maintenance of normal speech and in the rehabilitation of disordered speech.

It is unrealistic and perhaps unwarranted to expect the investigator, who studies sensory phenomena in their totality, and the neurophysiologist, who becomes involved with sensation at a cellular level, to view oral sensation and perception from the same perspective. As Jerge (1967) has pointed out, however, eventually workers studying the problem at those different levels must reconcile their data, and observations of all types must intertwine to form a complete and accurate picture.

Jerge (1967) further notes that since research in sensory physiology has demonstrated that the central nervous system is capable of modifying, even at the level of the primary receptor, the quality of information admitted for subsequent transmission, the role of receptor inhibition in the trigeminal system must be clarified. Also, the importance of the reticular formation in oral sensation should be stressed, as it is well known that it has a profound influence on transmission through sensory relay nuclei. Attempts also should be made to specify the actual neurophysiological mechanism by which observed sensory events take place.

Inasmuch as sensory networks are capable of undergoing and, in fact, do undergo structural changes in response to long-term changes in level or quality of impinging stimuli and since sensation and perception as phenomena have a learning and experience component, the plasticity of the nervous system almost certainly will become a promising subject of investigation by sensory physiologists and rehabilitation specialists in the future.

The factors of retention, anatomical maturation and motor development that are thought to be critical for the development of oral discrimination abilities also are said to underlie the processes of speech. It is hoped that in the future investigators will ask whether sensory discrimination abilities and speech development exist in a cause-effect relationship or whether they both are related to more general factors such as neurological maturation or perceptual skill development. If the cause-effect hypothesis is accepted, oral sensory disturbances can be considered as a new etiologic entity for defects of articulation, and ways of compensating for such disturbed input channels should be sought.

In such future work we must explore rehabilitation approaches that further develop prosthetic devices such as those described by Grossman and Bosma (1963) which may assist patients in compensating for sensory deficits. Also, efforts must be directed at identifying pharmacologic agents that might promote the discrimination process. If, as noted earlier, sensation and perception have a learning and experiential foundation, then Magoun's (1967) comments on recent studies of the facilitation of learning by such neuronal stimulants as caffeine, strychnine and picrotoxin may be relevant to persons demonstrating speech disorders etiologically based on sensory-system dysfunctioning.

A number of questions about the nature of speech therapy for persons with oral sensory disturbances must be investigated also. Should training be aimed at developing the use of input channels for speech monitoring that might serve in lieu of the disturbed channel (Chase, 1967), or should the tactile-kinesthetic channel be used regardless of its level of functioning? If it can be demonstrated that speech proficiency and oral discrimination ability are interdependent skills, then the value of teaching oral discrimination tasks as a requisite (or prerequisite) for conventional therapy should be explored. An attempt at this form of therapy has been reported by Shelton and his associates (1970). Their efforts to teach discrimination of palatal movements have not at all been encouraging but, at this stage of experimentation, should not dissuade future research efforts in this general direction.

The tasks we use to measure oral discrimination abilities also must be studied further. Such research must be directed toward the delineation of types and levels of sensory functioning called for by tasks of oral form-recognition and discrimination. It is only when these questions can be answered that an understanding of the significance of this deficit in pathological speakers can be attained. In this respect it should be noted that some excellent suggestions for research have been proposed (Shelton, Arndt and

Hetherington, 1967).

With reference to better understanding the effects on speech of disturbed oral sensation, techniques of physiologic articulatory phonetics should be employed to specify further the exact nature of articulatory changes which occur. Such techniques might include pressure and flow measures, cineradiographic and motion picture observations and electromyography. To illustrate further the need for technique development we need only look at the limitations placed upon the interpretation of nerve-block experiment results by our inability to adequately test the potential motor effects of anesthetizing drugs. Harris (1970) notes that a subject studied in her laboratory by EMG procedures demonstrated mylohyoid paralysis after a nerve-block injection. While EMG results of the type reported by Harris are important in studying motor functioning, they do not provide a clear method for determining whether the atypical EMG pattern is truly reflective of a motor system paralysis or whether the patient exhibits abnormal motor activity (as demonstrated in EMG recordings) because of a sensory deficit. Although this problem may be dealt with by direct neural stimulation techniques, such approaches have not found common use in studies of the speech musculature. Future research must develop tests that will allow for the clear determination of the level at which the speech system fails in different types of communicative disorders.

By way of summary, the ability to differentiate between normal-speaking and speech-disordered persons on the basis of information gained through sensory testing is significant both from an applied and a theoretic point of view. Evidence supporting the view that normal speech is reflected in orosensory functioning argues for the acceptance of a speech-production model that incorporates some servomechanical features and for a variety of therapeutic practices that are compatible with such a model. Any theorizing about the processes of speech and language development and their maintenance must take into account the sensory mechanisms underlying articulatory activity (Ringel *et al.*, 1970).

REFERENCES

Addis, Maureen: Oral perception: an evaluation of normal and defective speakers. Master's thesis, Purdue University, 1968.

Arndt, W. B., Elbert, Mary, and Shelton, R. L.: Standardization of a test of oral stereognosis. In J. F. Bosma (Ed.): Second Symposium on Oral Sensation and Perception. Springfield, Thomas, 1970.

Blom, S.: Afferent influences on tongue muscle activity. Acta Physiol Scand, 49:Suppl. 170, 1960.

Bosma, J. F.: A Syndrome of impairment in oral perception. In J. F. Bosma (Ed.): Symposium on Oral Sensation and Perception. Springfield, Thomas, 1967.

Chase, R. A.: Abnormalities in motor control secondary to congenital sensory defects. In J. F. Bosma (Ed.): Symposium on Oral Sensation and Perception. Springfield, Thomas, 1967.

Cooper, Sybil: Muscle spindles in the intrinsic muscles of the human tongue. J Physiol, 122:193-202, 1953.

Fairbanks, G.: Systematic research in experimental phonetics: 1. A theory of the speech mechanism as a servosystem. J Speech Hear Disord, 19:133-199, 1954.

Fucci, D. J.: Oral vibro-tactile perception: An evaluation of normal and defective speakers. Doctoral dissertation, Purdue University, 1968.

Gammon, S. A., Smith, P., Daniloff, R., Kim, C.: Articulation and stress/juncture production under oral anesthetization and masking. J Speech Hear Res, 14:271-282, 1971.

Grossman, R. C., and Bosma, J. F.: Experimental oral sensory prosthesis. J Dent Res, 42:891, 1963.

Grossman, R. C., and Hattis, Barbara: Oral mucosal sensory innervation and sensory experience. In J. F. Bosma (Ed.): Symposium on Oral Sensation and Perception. Springfield, Thomas, 1967.

Grossman, R. C., Hattis, B. F., and Ringel, R. L.: Oral tactile experience. Arch Oral Biol, 10:691-705, 1965.

Hardy, J. C.: Development of neuromuscular systems underlying speech production. Speech and the Dentofacial Complex: The State of the Art. ASHA Reports #5, 49-68, 1970.

Harris, Katherine S.: Physiological measures of speech movements: EMG and fiberoptic studies. Speech and the Dentofacial Complex: The State of the Art, ASHA Reports #5, 271-283, 1970.

Henja, R. F.: A study of the role of kinesthetic cues in stuttering. Paper presented at the Annual Convention of the American Speech and Hearing Association, New York, 1962.

Henke, W.: Preliminaries to speech synthesis based upon an articulatory model. Paper presented at the Conference on Speech Communications and Processing, Cambridge, 1967.

Hochberg, I., and Kabcenell, J.: Oral stereognosis in normal and cleft-palate individuals. Cleft Palate J, 4:47-57, 1967.

Jerge, C. R.: The neural substratum of oral sensation. In J. F. Bosma (Ed.): Symposium on Oral Sensation and Perception. Springfield, Thomas, 1967.

Kawamura, Y.: Neuromuscular mechanisms of jaw and tongue movement. J Am Dent Assoc, 62:545-551, 1961.

Kawamura, Y.: Oral physiology and clinical dentistry. J Dent Educ, 29:179-185, 1965.

Kirchner, J., and Wyke, B.: Afferent discharges from laryngeal articular mechanorecptors. Nature, 205:86, 1965.

Ladefoged, P.: Three Areas of Experimental Phonetics. London, Oxford University Press, 1967.

Lane, J.: A motor theory of speech perceptions: A critical review. Psychol Rev, 72:275-309, 1965.

Liberman, A. M.: Some results of research on speech perception. J Acoust Soc Am, 29:117-123, 1957.

Liberman, A. M., Harris, Katherine, Eimas, P., Lisker, L., and Bastian, J.: An effect of learning on speech perception: The discrimination of durations of silence with and without phonemic significance. Lang Speech, 4:175-195, 1961.

Locke, J. L.: Oral perception and articulation learning. Percept Mot Skills, 26:1259-1264, 1968.

McCall, G. N., and Kirkley, D., Jr.: An approach to the measurement of thresholds of tactile sensitivity in the oral and perioral regions of the body. Paper presented at the Annual Convention of the American Speech and Hearing Association, Chicago, 1967.

McCroskey, R. L., Jr.: The relative contribution of auditory and tactile cues to certain aspects of speech. S Speech J, 24:84-90, 1958.

McCroskey, R. L., Corley, N. W., and Jackson, G.: Some effects of disrupted tactile cues upon the production of consonants. S Speech J, 25:55-60, 1959.

McDonald, E. T., and Aungst, L. F.: Studies in oral sensorimotor function. In J. F. Bosma (Ed.): Symposium on Oral Sensation and Perception. Springfield, Thomas, 1967.

McDonald, E. T., and Aungst, L. F.: Apparent independence of oral sensory functions and articulation proficiency. In J. F. Bosma (Ed.): Second Symposium on Oral Sensation and Perception. Springfield, Thomas, 1970.

MacNeilage, D. F.: Motor control of serial ordering of speech. Psychol Rev, 77:182-196, 1970.

Magoun, J. W.: Lacunae and research approaches to them. In C. H. Millikan and F. L. Darley (Eds.): Brain Mechanisms Underlying Speech and Language. New York, Grune and Stratton, 1967.

Mason, R. M.: Studies of oral perception involving subjects with alterations in anatomy and physiology. In J. R. Bosma (Ed.): Symposium on Oral Sensation and Perception. Springfield, Thomas, 1967.

Matthews, P. B. C.: Muscle spindles and their motor control. Physiol Rev, 44:219-287, 1964.

Melzack, R., and Wall, P.: On the nature of cutaneous sensory mechanisms.

Brain, 85:331-356, 1962.

Moser, H., LaGourgue, J. R., and Class, Lois: Studies of oral stereognosis in normal, blind and deaf subjects. In J. F. Bosma (Ed.): Symposium on Oral Sensation and Perception. Springfield, Thomas, 1967.

Paillard, J.: The patterning of skilled movement. In J. Field, H. W. Magoun, and V. E. Hall (Eds.): Neurophysiology. Washington, D. C., Amer. Physiol. Soc., 1960, vol. III.

Perkell, J. S.: Physiology of Speech Production: Results and Implications of a Quantitative Cineradiographic Study. Cambridge, MIT Press, 1969.

Ringel, R. L.: Some effects of tactile and auditory alternations on speech output. Doctoral dissertation, Purdue University, 1962.

Ringel, R. L.: Oral region two-point discrimination in normal and myopathic subjects. In J. F. Bosma (Ed.): Second Symposium on Oral Sensation and Perception. Springfield, Thomas, 1970.

Ringel, R. L., Burk, K. W., and Scott, Cheryl M.: Tactile perception: Form discrimination in the mouth. Br J Disord Commun, 3:150-155, 1968.

Ringel, R. L., and Ewanowski, S. J.: Oral perception: 1. Two-point discrimination. J. Speech Hearing Res., 8:389-398, 1965.

Ringel, R. L., and Fletcher, Hilary: Oral perception: III. Texture discrimination. J Speech Hear Res, 10:642-649, 1967.

Ringel, R. L., House, A. S., Burk, K. W., Dolinsky, J. P., and Scott, Cheryl M.: Some relations between oral sensory discrimination and articulatory aspects of speech production. J Speech Hear Disord, 35:3-11, 1970.

Ringel, R. L., and Steer, M. D.: Some effects of tactile and auditory alterations on speech output. J Speech Hear Res, 6:369-378, 1963.

Rootes, T. P., and MacNeilage, P. F.: Some speech perception and production tests of a patient with impairment in somesthetic perception and motor function. In J. F. Bosma (Ed.): Symposium on Oral Sensation and Perception. Springfield, Thomas, 1967.

Rose, J. E., and Mountcastle, V. B.: Touch and kinesthesis. In J. Field, H. W. Magoun, and V. E. Hall (Eds.): Neurophysiology. Washington, D. C.: Amer. Physiol. Soc., 1969, vol. I.

Rutherford, D., and McCall, G.: Testing oral sensation and perception in persons with dysarthria. In J. F. Bosma (Ed.): Symposium on Oral Sensation and Perception. Springfield, Thomas, 1967.

Schliesser, H. F.: Restricted motility of the speech articulators and selected sensory discriminative modalities of speech defective spastic hemiplegic children. Doctoral dissertation, University of Iowa, 1965.

Schliesser, H. F., and Coleman, R. O.: Effectiveness of certain procedures of alteration of auditory and oral tactile sensations for speech. Percept Mot Skills, 26:275-281, 1968.

Scott, C. M., and Ringel, R. L.: Articulation without oral sensory control. J Speech Hear Res, 14:804-818, 1971.

Scott, C. M., and Ringel, R. L.: The effects of motor and sensory disruptions on speech: A description of articulation. J Speech Hear Res, 14:819-828, 1971.

Shelton, R. L.: Oral sensory function in speech production. In W. C. Grass, S. W. Rosenstein, and K. R. Bzoch (Eds.): Cleft Lip and Palate. Little, Brown (in press).

Shelton, R. L., Arndt, W. B., and Hetherington, J. J.: Testing oral stereognosis. In J. F. Bosma (Ed.): Second Symposium on Oral Sensation and Perception. Springfield, Thomas, 1970.

Shelton, R. L., Knox, A. W., Elbert, Mary, and Johnson, T. S.: Palate awareness and non-speech voluntary palate movement. In J. F. Bosma (Ed.): Second Symposium on Oral Sensation and Perception. Springfield, Thomas, 1970.

Shewchuk, L., and Zubek, J.: Discriminatory ability of various skin areas as measured by a technique of intermittent stimulation. Can J Psychol, 14:244-248, 1960.

Silverman, S.: Oral Physiology, St. Louis, Mosby, 1961.

Sinclair, D.: Cutaneous sensation and the doctrine of specific energy. Brain, 78:583-614, 1955.

Solomon, B.: The relation of oral sensation and perception to chewing, drinking and articulation in athetoid children and adults. Doctoral dissertation, Pennsylvania State University, August, 1965.

Thompson, R. C.: The effects of oral sensory disruption upon oral stereognosis and articulation. Paper presented at the Annual Convention of the American Speech and Hearing Association, Chicago, 1969.

Weber, B. A.: Effect of high level masking and anesthetization of oral structures upon articulatory proficiency and voice characteristics of normal speakers. Master's thesis, Pennsylvania State University, 1961.

Weinberg, B., Lyons, Sister M. J., and Liss, Gail M.: Studies of oral, manual and visual form identification skills in children and adults. In J. F. Bosma (Ed.): Second Symposium on Oral Sensation and Perception. Springfield, Thomas, 1970.

Weiss, C. E.: The effects of disrupted lingua-palatal taction on physiologic parameters of articulation. J Comm Dis, 2:312-321, 1969.

Wyke, B.: Recent advances in the neurology of phonation: Reflex mechanisms in the larynx. Br J Disord Commun, 2:2-14, 1967.

CHAPTER III

DEVELOPMENTAL ASPECTS
OF ARTICULATION

MILDRED C. TEMPLIN

$\int$MASTERY of the phonemic system is an integral part of a child's development of language. The phonemes provide the basic building blocks for the words of the language, and these, in turn, are an essential part of the grammatical system. During the period of language acquisition which essentially covers the preschool and early school years, the child recognizes the symbolic function of language, establishes the rudiments of the grammar of the language of his community and masters the phonemic system. The child will, throughout life, continue to develop elaborations and subtle refinements of the grammar, add new words to his vocabulary and delineate more functions of language usage. Articulation deals with the production of the phonemes of the language. Adequate articulation is achieved by most children when they are seven or eight years of age. Those comparatively few children who have not mastered it by this age are potential candidates for speech therapy.

A number of factors obviously are associated with a child's mastery of the perception and production of the phonemes: motor control of the organs of phonation and articulation involved in their production; skill in the recognition of a variety of acoustic, kinesthetic, tactual and visual cues that may contrast sounds; and substantial experience with language usage. Although

NOTE: The longitudinal study reported in this chapter was supported by the United States Office of Education through the Cooperative Research Program and the Research, Development and Demonstration Center in Education of Handicapped Children, University of Minnesota.

all of these are recognized as associated with the development of the mastery of phonemes, one factor is frequently emphasized over another according to the particular language interest of the theorist or researcher.

A major barrier to understanding the early articulation development of children is that the descriptive accounts of what actually occurs are inadequate. This deficiency has been emphasized repeatedly in current, and recognized in older, literature (for example, Lewis, 1936; Siegel, 1964; Weir, 1967; McNeill, 1970; and Menyuk, 1971). Reasons for this deficiency are complex but are related primarily to the pervasive and painstaking nature of the problems associated with obtaining such data. There is a need, too, for more study of the interrelationship among the various language behaviors. Weir, after studying the grammatical, phonemic and intonational patterns of her own children, emphasized the possible importance of information on intonational patterns as offering relevant clues to understanding the relationship between learning syntax and learning phonology.

A discussion of articulation development must, of necessity, be only a general guide, since the course of development of individual children varies considerably. However, general trends of development have long been accepted in developmental psychology. Sequences of locomotor, cognitive and social development are almost universally recognized. Recently Brown (1968) pointed out that the sequence of grammatical control was essentially similar for Adam, Eve and Sarah, the three children he has been studying, but the rate of acquisition of adequate grammars varied among the children.

A distinction is made between the prelanguage and the language periods. During the prelanguage period the child responds to language, utters sounds and series of sounds with different intonation, but does not use these utterances in actual verbal communication. Nevertheless, he is immersed in a verbal environment which reinforces the functions of language, discriminates meaning on the basis of phonemes, morphemes, words and grammatical structures and provides experiences that delineate content for communication. During the language period the child uses verbal utterances for meaningful communication. Not until this occurs can the development of the use of phonemes, grammar and syntax be traced.

The prelanguage and language periods are not sharply separated, since they represent categories within the process of language development. It is difficult to determine when a child first uses the utterance of either a dictionary item or an esoteric combination of sounds as a meaningful word. The identification of the point at which a shift from the prelanguage to the language period occurs is far less important than the recognition of the shift to meaningful speech.

Problems associated with the determination of when a functional word is uttered by the child are clearly pointed up in a summary of the literature on the age of use of first word (Darley and Winitz, 1961). Mothers in one study reported the first word about five months earlier than the experimenters who visited the home periodically (Shirley, 1936). Mothers may have identified a word earlier because they read meaning into the early utterances of their children. Or they may have heard the word earlier because they were with their children for longer periods of time and thus were more likely to be present when an infrequent early word was uttered. In the long run, the parent is probably the best judge of when a child actually begins to use words, that is, to talk.

At the beginning of the language period a child may be using only one or two words. The number of different words that he uses will most probably increase very slowly for several months. Even when the young child has begun to use two-word and three-word sentences, he will probably still continue to use some non-language utterances that can be interpreted essentially only as nonsense or gibberish.

A look at vocalization during the prelanguage period indicates that, apart from the crying, fussing, belching and other organic sounds, the infant, during the first half year of life, produces sounds that to the listener sound like phonemes. These cooing sounds are usually described as primarily vocalic, but some consonant sounds do appear. Toward the latter half of the first year of life, babbling tends to replace cooing. Babbling usually refers to the utterances of the infant which give the impression of duplicative syllables that are frequently uttered with intonations resembling those of the language of the child's community. While these utterances may vaguely resemble speech acoustically, they are not attached to any consistent cognitive meaning.

There is no real agreement on the relation between a child's cooing and babbling and between his babbling and early speech. Siegel (1969) has recently discussed the relation between cooing and babbling and points out, that while it is recognized that the vocalizations of infants during babbling more nearly approximate the phonemes of the language of the child's community than those made during cooing, the process that best characterizes this change is not clear. Two theories are proposed: (1) A *contraction* theory which holds that as speech develops from the large number of sounds uttered by the young child, inappropriate sounds are deleted and appropriate ones retained and (2) an *expansion* theory which holds that a young child's repertoire of speech sounds is initially very limited and that it increases as he matures. It is probable that in children's early utterances many sounds may be relatively ambiguous productions and that the development of an adult repertoire of sounds involves "both the strengthening of certain sounds to the exclusion of others (contraction) and the shaping of more amorphous sounds into acceptable productions (a kind of expansion)" (Siegel, 1969, p. 5). However, of special interest is the fact that sufficient descriptive data to support either point of view are lacking. Available data do suggest that by the time the child has shifted to the babbling stage, the patterns of the language of the child's community have become apparent. For example, Irwin has indicated that the / ? / is not heard in the utterances of Midwestern infants after about six months, and Weir suggests that at six to seven months the utterances of a Chinese infant could be distinguished from those of an American and Russian infant.

The role of babbling in the development of early speech is also disputed. There is agreement that during the period of babbling, the utterances of children have a superficial resemblance to speech, but real language is not present. Some hold that there is no significant relationship between the two periods, and others consider them necessary parts of a continuous process of development. Over these periods, too, the need of accurate descriptions of the vocal performance of children is apparent.

Those who consider babbling and speech to be unrelated have emphasized, primarily, the development of the phoneme system.

They have postulated a period of silence preceding the initiation of speech (McNeill, 1970). The first language of children has a very restricted vocabulary and is situation bound. The grammatical and semantic restrictions of the child's early utterances may also restrict the range of phonemes necessary for the child to communicate at this level. Children utter many more recognizable sound which to a listener resembles the phoneme. The production example, a child may produce (kaka) in babbling but say /te/ for /kek/ in his early speech. The use of the appropriate phoneme in a word presents a different task from the mere production of a sound which to a listener resenbles the phoneme. The production of the sound in a word involves not only motor control, but perceptual discrimination and cognitive processing, whereas the babbling utterance may be largely a sensori-motor function. The former is an intentional utterance and the latter may be accidental. It is possible that certain sounds are not used in words because they do not fit into the child's level of phonemic development, and not because he cannot perceive or articulate them.

Those who look upon the babbling period as an important link in the development of early speech do not emphasize phonemic development, per se, but consider babbling as a time in which factors necessary for speech are developed and practiced. A number of different factors may be emphasized—for example, the cumulative experience gained in sound production, the establishment of intonation patterns and the diversification of use and the enjoyment of vocalization. Fry (1967), for example, sees the babbling stage as making two important contributions to early language: the first in the basic discovery of the possibilities inherent in the use of the mechanisms involved in phonation and articulation, and the second in the establishment of the auditory feedback loop by which motor activity and auditory impressions are linked together for the child. Through these the child gains control of the muscular systems used in speech and not only learns the acoustic result of making certain movements, but discovers how to make the movements again and again in order to produce essentially the same acoustic results.

Several decades ago, Lewis (1936) based his discussion of how speech begins in children on a collation of his own careful observations and the available observations of others. He believed that the development of a child's language could only be fully understood in the light of his earliest utterances and that these needed to be interpreted in relation to the situation in which they occurred. For him observation of characteristics of the child's utterances, of the child's responsiveness to speech and the situation in which these occurred were necessary components in the investigation of infant speech. He related the place of articulation of sounds uttered in the early months of life to the state of comfort or discomfort of the child. He considered babbling the important time for the beginning of the esthetic use of language.

Among the many contributions of Lewis, his concept of speech as a complex of phonetic and intonational patterns is of great importance today when interest in the prosodic features of young children's utterances is rising. In his discussion of the interrelationship he distinguishes a sequence of development. At an early age children distinguish between expressive and representational intonation. In the former, the rhythm, stress and pitch of the utterance express the emotional state of the speaker. In the latter, they represent the situation, as, for example, when *tick-tock* is spoken in time with a clock. When both phonetic form and intonational patterns have become effective for the child, the intonational pattern dominates his response. As the child develops functional speech, however, the phonemic system becomes dominant. Nevertheless, the function of the intonational pattern, while it is considerably reduced, does not disappear.

It has been stated that a child understands language before he uses it, but this statement is too general to be of much help in understanding the role of the child's perception of language in his learning of it. In a summary and discussion of the role of perception of language during the prelanguage and the early language periods, Friedlander (1970) deplored the sparcity of such research. In the twenties and thirties the responsiveness of infants to gross auditory stimuli composed of a variety of human and non-human noises was systematically studied. Recently a variety of studies aimed at delineating the child's responsiveness to specific phonemes and characteristics of speech and language have been undertaken. There is no doubt that even as neonates, children respond to auditory stimuli and that within the first months of life they respond differentially to selected phonemes, to differences in familiar and unfamiliar voices and to different qualities of voice. Increasing concern for exploring the interaction between perception and production of language should result in substantial gains in knowledge within the foreseeable future.

A number of developmental and normative studies have attempted to describe utterances of children as phonemes perceived by listeners across the prelanguage and language periods. While there is substantial agreement in general aspects of the phonemic development, a specific sequence of phonemes is not described.

Until the work of Irwin (1946) diary records of individual children provided almost all of the available descriptions at the prelanguage period. He and his associates in broad phonemic transcription of the International Phonetic Alphabet transcribed the phonemes of English that they recognized in the utterances of 95 infants. Utterances were transcribed during thirty breath groups obtained at two-month intervals from birth to about thirty months of age. Some 35 children were observed throughout. Before the end of this period children are using language meaningfully.

During the language period a number of descriptive studies have been carried on (Wellman, 1936; Templin, 1957; Snow, 1963). The most recent and extensive is the writer's normative study that was based on the articulation of 480 children selected to form a representative sample according to their fathers' occupations. The sixty subjects who made up each age sample at half-year intervals from three to five years and from six to eight years were tested within one month of their designated ages. A more extensive normative study is currently under way (Hull, 1971).

The following brief summary of the phonemes recognized in children's utterances relies heavily upon the works of Irwin and Templin. Utterances of the front vowels and the back consonants predominate during the first year. During the second year, the back vowels and front consonants increase in frequency. By the end of the first year, about three-fourths of the vowels and about one-third of the consonants of English are recognizable. By two-and-a-half years, practically all of the vowels and about two-thirds of the consonants are present.

During the first months of life, sibilant sounds and those made in the velar and glottal positions account for a large proportion of the sounds uttered. There is a gradual change, however, so that the distribution of sounds both by type and position uttered by two-and-a-half year olds approximates those used by adults. The bilabial sounds, such as the /m/ and /b/, appear frequently in children's first words, although they are not common among the early vocalizations of the prelanguage period.

Most children produce vowels and nasals appropriately and accurately in words by the age of three. Stops are produced correctly at an earlier age than fricatives. It is not until seven or eight years of age that practically all children attain adequate articulation in a testing situation. Boys tend to reach this level about six months to a year later than girls. However this difference is psychologically unimportant because it occurs at a time when the level of achievement for boys and girls, as a whole, is already high.

The frequency and kind of developmental consonant misarticulations vary with the particular sounds and their positions in a syllable. Sounds at the beginnings of syllables are produced correctly at an earlier age than those at the end of syllables. About 90 per cent of the misarticulations of children involve the substitution of either another English phoneme or of a distorted approximation. The proportion of these substitutions and distortions among misarticulations is relatively constant from age to age. The omission of a sound is a much less common deviation. It decreases substantially with age and is usually associated with immature articulation. Snow has provided useful information on the specific substitutions of *normal* first grade children who misarticulate the phonemes of English in the initial, medial and final positions of words.

The last ten consonant sounds acquired developmentally according to Templin's cross-sectional data are the most frequent misarticulations of *normal* five- to nine-year-olds (Wepman and

Morency, 1963). Misarticulations of these sounds have been termed *age appropriate,* and the substitutions and distortions of them decrease dramatically during the first three years in school. Profiles of the productions of these age-appropriate sounds differentiate among children with misarticulations resulting from developmental lag, cleft palate and mental retardation. They do not differentiate between children with normal articulation and those classified as lagging in development according to Wepman. In Templin's longitudinal study discussed later, the proportion of these sounds misarticulated is being explored as a possible predictor of later articulation.

Children of three and four years are able to recognize the combinations of phonemes which appear and do not appear in English words (Messer, 1967). Furthermore, the substitutions that occur in their pronunciations of combinations of sounds that would not occur in English words, move these combinations in the direction of sound clusters acceptable in English words. Thus, for example, / ʃpeln/ is frequently reproduced as /speln/, and /tʃ1ʌ f/ as /ʃ1ʌ f/.

A few studies have appeared which suggest that children who lack mastery of the production of the sound system may also exhibit inadequacies in their use of syntax. Thus children from three to six years (Menyuk, 1964; Shriner *et al.,* 1969) with speech described as *infantile* or as at least one standard deviation below the mean for their age on the *Templin-Darly Tests of Articulation* were found to use restricted syntactical forms and essentially underdeveloped syntax on a number of dimensions. Some data from the writer's longitudinal study discussed later also supports this in relation to articulation and the application of morphological rules in kindergarten, first and second grade.

In 1941 Jakobson proposed that the development of the phoneme system be looked at in terms of the acquisition of sound categories rather than of the acquisition of specific phonemes. This important work in which the theory of distinctive features was set forth has only recently been translated into English (1968). It considers speech sounds as composed of bundles of both articulatory and acoustic attributes or features. Some thirteen features identified include voicing, nasality, continuancy, gravity, stridency, etc. A matrix can be prepared for each phoneme indicating whether each feature is significant (+) for the phoneme, or whether it is absent from the phoneme and therefore not significant (-) for it. For any two sounds the matrices of features will differ in at least one feature, and a single feature may be shared by many sounds. Comparison of patterns within the feature matrices for the phonemes of English permits grouping of sounds on the basis of the presence or absence of specific distinctive features. These groupings cut across the traditional classifications of phonemes according to nasals, stops, etc

Jakobson proposed that the development of the phoneme system is the result of a progressive differentiation of maximal contrasts. Thus the child first differentiates between those pairs of sounds in which there is the least overlap among the significant (+) distinctive features, i.e. the grossest or maximal contrast is the first learned. As development progresses, contrasts are continued to be made between features that are maximally different. Thus, for example, the vowel-consonant contrast (usually described as initially between /a/ and /p/) is probably the earliest contrast achieved by all children and is followed by the stop-continuant contrasts in place of articulation (e.g. labial versus dental, stops /p/ versus /t/ or nasals /m/ versus /n/), contrasts in voicing (e.g., /p/ versus /b/), etc. For the most part, these contrasts have been verified not upon empirical data gathered for the purpose, but upon the reexamination of phonemic descriptive data such as previously described.

Distinctive feature theory permits the consideration of the development of the phoneme system in terms of rules of phonology that the child has established. It also permits the study of the development of phonology across languages because contrasts achieved, rather than phonemes produced, are considered. Since the maximum contrasts to be discriminated are similar in all languages, distinctive feature theory may be a key in the search for phonological universals.

It is interesting that the concept of distinctive features has been so slow to have a major impact on the study of sound development and deviation. Twenty years ago, Leopold (1953) recognized it as "epoch making" and applied it to his observations of the utterances of his daughter. For a long time, however, it was not used in empirical research.

Some years ago a number of studies looked at misarticulations in terms of attributes of voicing, place and manner of articulation. For example, Prins (1962) described misarticulations of children between three and six in terms of the number of these three attributes that varied from the expected phoneme. Snow (1964) has suggested that the substitutions of normally speaking first graders frequently match the expected phoneme on manner of articulation. These studies, however, looked only at a few specific attributes in a somewhat static fashion.

Attempts are being made to determine empirically the contrasts that are essential for the English phonemic system, as well as the sequence in which the distinctive feature contrasts appear developmentally. All of the distinct features identified have not been included in these attempts, and different features have been considered by various investigators. On the whole, at present, solid data are only beginning to appear. As suggested by Winitz in Chapter 5, the concept of distinctive features may well have an increasing influence on the study of articulation deviation and projected therapy in the years ahead.

The impact of the concept of generative grammar (Chomsky, 1957) is now becoming apparent in the study of the child's articulation of the phoneme system of the language. This concept changes the emphasis and the options of interpretation of the child's performance. A sound production by the child is then considered not as an incident, per se, but as an expression of a phonological rule of the child. Performance and understanding are thus linked. Crocker (1969) has constructed a theoretical linguistic model to represent the development of children's linguistic competence in terms of rules for the combination of distinctive features. The rules presented in the model seem to specify effectively the developmental progression from general to more specified sound usage observed in children. The author emphasizes that though the model appears to be valid, in order for it to be useful it must be verified against a wide range of speech performance in children.

The few instances in which misarticulations of children have been analyzed for generative phonological rules have suggested both the value of the approach and the necessity for its further study. Compton (1970) emphasized that the misarticulations of children should be looked upon as an expression of their phonological rules. He has analyzed the articulation of two children and found that their misarticulations are systematic when measured against their own phonological rules. In another study, McReynolds and Huston (1971) examined the utterances of ten children with severe misarticulation problems, both according to the specific phonemes misarticulated and the 13 distinctive features maintained by the children in comparison with the features demanded by the English phoneme system. The value of the distinctive feature analysis was shown in that the children were consistent in their feature errors and, as Compton had also found, that one or two features could account for the misarticulation of several phonemes. However, two patterns of feature errors emerged. In one, the child was able to produce the various features, but his rules for applying them differed from the phonological rules of English. In the other, misarticulation could be described as including omission of one or two features as well as the incorrect production of some features.

Throughout this discussion, the phoneme, that long-standing primary unit of language learning, has been considered. In recent years, a number of important concepts have begun to redefine our approach to articulation. Of these, only the concepts of generative grammar and distinctive features theory have been included. Omission of such concepts as the syllable as the basic unit of language learning, of coarticulation and of the motor theory of language learning was dictated by space constraints and not by any implication of their lack of significance.

A LONGITUDINAL STUDY

For a number of years the writer has been engaged in a longitudinal study of articulation that deals directly with daily tasks of public school speech clinicians. It is concerned with the development of articulation in the early school years and attempts to identify factors that are associated with later achievement of adequate or inadequate articulation. How, really, can we define an articulation deviation at a time when satisfactory articulation is not yet attained by many children who will later achieve it? Which children should be given speech therapy? Do we, or can we, really know which children will spontaneously achieve adequate articulation? When the writer was a student in speech pathology in the thirties these were important, unanswered questions, and they still are.

Public school clinicians must continuously make decisions that diagnose articulation deviations and determine therapy procedures. These decisions reflect the best knowledge, experience and judgment of each clinician. Any research study can be important to these decisions, if the speech clinician finds it relevant. Some research is more likely to be directly meaningful to speech clinicians, however, merely because the problem is studied in terms of hypotheses or questions that are related to tasks of public school speech clinicians. This longitudinal study of articulation is such an investigation. However, it will not be discussed as a research project, per se. Rather, the emphasis will be on aspects of the problem, the design, the procedure and some tentative results that have implications for public school speech clinicians. Before this can be done, a very brief overview of the study is needed.

In this study, 435 children representing a wide range of articulation adequacy have been tested at eleven six-month intervals between pre-kindergarten and the end of fourth grade and will again be tested when the subjects are in eleventh grade. They were selected for longitudinal study from 1,500 children whose articulation was first tested in both spontaneous and imitative utterances during the spring before they entered kindergarten. They were assigned to study samples on the basis of characteristics of articulation that seemed most likely to be related to later defective articulation: divergence between their picture and imitative articulation test scores, their number of misarticulations and their specific misarticulations. No subject assigned to study samples had any known organic problem related to articulation. With few exceptions the samples included at least 25 boys or 25 girls. Boys and girls were selected on their own distributions of articulation scores.

The samples selected are as follows. One *shift sample* was made up of children whose percentage of spontaneous and imitative articulation scores obtained at the same test session differed by at least four McCall T-Score points. From the children whose articulation scores were essentially the same whether obtained with or without an aural model, imitation articulation scores were used to select five percentile samples according to the total number of misarticulations and three phoneme samples according to the specific phonemes misarticulated. Total imitation articulation test scores of subjects in the five *percentile samples* clustered about the 7th, 15th, 30th, 50th and 98th percentiles of the kindergarten distributions of such scores for each sex. According to cross-sectional norms (Templin, 1957), the articulation of the children in the 7th percentile samples resembled that of three-and-a-half-year-olds, and the articulation of those in the 98th percentile samples resembled that of seven- or eight-year-olds. Articulation of children in the 50th percentile samples resembled that of five- to six-year-old children. These were considered built-in normative samples since their articulation was typical of kindergarten-aged children. Three *phoneme samples* were selected in which the /r/, /l/ or /s/ phoneme was the single major misarticulation. For example, to be included in the /s/-phoneme sample, it was necessary that a child misarticulate at least five-sixths of his utterances of /s/ and less than one-sixth of those of /r/ or /l/.

Articulation has been assessed each spring and fall between pre-kindergarten and the end of fourth grade by a number of different measures and will be again at the end of the eleventh grade. At every session, production of the consonants of English and of six consonant clusters containing /r/, /l/ and /s/ phonemes was evaluated in words elicited both by pictures and repeated after the examiner. With only one exception (the / ʒ / as in *treasure)* the initial or final consonant in the syllable was also the initial or final sound in an English word. Other frequently-used articulation measures evaluated productions of consonant singles in nonsense words, and a substantial number of consonant clusters in the initial or final positions within words. At selected sessions, tests were given the children in the general areas of speech, reading, spelling, language, auditory and visual stimuli, personality, intelligence and motor skills. On some of these, the articulation of the responses was transcribed. The longitudinal study samples and all the tests used through fourth grade have been described in detail elsewhere (Templin, 1967).

The analyses planned and partially completed include: (1) Inter-sample comparisons of the development of articulation and its relation to nonarticulation performance. (2) Intra-sample comparisons of those children who do and do not achieve adequate articulation at second, third or fourth grade in an attempt to identify factors which may be able to differentiate them at the lower grades. (3) Comparison of the characteristics and patterns of development of pairs of individual children matched with similar articulation performance in kindergarten but only one of whom achieves adequate articulation in the later grades.

A few years ago a representative sample of nearly 2,000 public school speech clinicians identified the need for development of better criteria for selection of primary-grade children for remedial speech programs and the collection of longitudinal data on speech (Pronovost *et al.,* 1969). The implication of these problems is far-reaching because of the large numbers of children enrolled in speech therapy in the public schools. Estimates for the 1966 enrollment by the National Center of Educational Statistics indicate that of 1,794,000 children enrolled in special programs for children with speech, visual, auditory, intellectual, physical and emotional impairments, some 989,500 were speech impaired (Mackie, 1969). Over 80 per cent of the case load of public school speech clinicians is made up of children with articulation impairments (Bingham *et al.,* 1961).

There is not a great deal of research on prediction. Even though there has been an increase during the past decade, the surface of the problem has barely been scratched. Much of the research that has been done is to be found in single, isolated studies, that, for the most part, are quite insulated from one another. Only a few persons have intensively investigated the problem of prediction (see, for example, Van Riper, 1967; Wepman, 1967; and Pronovost, 1966). If basic information on the prediction of articulation is to be obtained, research in this area needs to be concerted, concentrated and continuing.

There are a number of reasons for the dearth of research on development and prediction. Speech clinicians most intimately concerned frequently do not have the necessary skills for such research. If they do, the pressures and goals of clinical work to which they are basically committed preclude such study or make it extremely difficult. In order for the study briefly described to have been carried out successfully, it was necessary that no speech therapy be given to the children in the public schools through the second grade. Persons concerned with the research design readily saw this. The public school speech supervisor understood it and was of great help in convincing principals and school administrators; parents readily brought their preschool children for testing even though they were told that no speech therapy would be given their children. The speech clinicians, however, while they understood the importance of trying to find ways of identifying those children with misarticulations who would and would not improve, were committed to rehabilitation and found it difficult to withhold therapy from children with known deficits.

Research on prediction and development is probably also scarce because longitudinal study is essential. It is not possible to obtain adequate information on developmental processes from cross-sectional data alone. However, longitudinal studies require a long-term commitment that may be difficult to live with. Such studies are bound methodologically to the past, regardless of the present interests of the investigator. There is no way to turn back the clock to obtain additional information or to use different techniques. Inevitably, subjects move, become ill and are lost to the sample. Not until the final testing can the sample be identified and the data analyzed. Days, weeks, months and years must pass if the growth of individual children is to be studied. The passage of time is the one essential variable of longitudinal study, and it cannot be controlled.

In a sense, the person engaged in longitudinal research is always out of phase with current interests. But current interests change, and, as Jones (1958) has pointed out, when an area seems most popular, interest in it has already crested. If one wants to know about the development of articulation or the prediction of its development in the same individuals, ultimately, there is no way to obtain the information other than by longitudinal study.

It is impossible to carry on a longitudinal study such as described here without the willing cooperation of many persons. Such cooperation was given by the administrators of the special education program in the public schools, the elementary school principals, the public school speech clinicians and the parents of the children. A letter describing the project and inviting participation in it was sent to the principals of the 84 city elementary schools over the writer's signature and that of the Director of Special Education. In response to the letter, all schools were made available for testing except ten that were unable to participate for such legitimate reasons as limited space, previous commitments to other studies and unique problems of scheduling children. However, because of limitations of time and project personnel, it was possible to test in only 45 of the available schools selected because it was possible for them to provide children, and space for testing them, at times that would fit into the schedules of the project examiners.

Fifteen hundred parents cooperated by bringing their prekindergarten children to the schools for articulation testing. The children brought in formed the pool of potential study subjects. The study had been described to the parents as attempting to discover if before youngsters entered kindergarten, those who would need speech therapy later could be identified. Parents were told that "children who speak well and those who speak very poorly are needed. Having your child's speech evaluated does not mean either that he should or that he will have speech correction. There is no therapy connected with the study. Bringing your child for speech evaluation, however, is an opportunity for you to help in obtaining information on the development of speech in children which should be useful in providing an even more efficient speech correction program for the . . . schools." Thus parents cooperated with no incentive of immediate reward and when the children selected for longitudinal study were in third grade, over 95 per cent of the parents filled in and returned a nine-page questionnaire.

The need for longitudinal data on articulation development is clearly brought out in this investigation. Because cross-sectional studies suggest that mature articulation is achieved by seven- to eight-year-old children, it was originally planned to terminate the longitudinal study when the children had finished the second grade. However, since a large number of children did not adequately produce the phonemes of English by the end of second grade, the study was continued through fourth and then extended to eleventh grade. At second grade, the articulation scores of only three of the approximately 60 children in the 7th percentile samples were at or above the median score for the 50th percentile sample for both sexes (the built-in normative samples). By the end of fourth grade, the mean articulation scores of the lowest percentile samples were approximately equal to that of the 50th percentile samples in kindergarten. Throughout the study, the scores of the 50th percentile samples quite closely resembled those of cross-sectional normative samples of the same age.

If the results of any investigation are to be used, the samples studied, as well as the methods used, must be carefully considered. Current emphasis on early identification of deviation strengthens the desirability of studying articulation in very young children. The constraints of reality, however, dictated that articulation be studied in children about to enter school and that it be continued during their early school years. While these children are too old for the study of the genesis of articulation, they are at an important age for public school speech clinicians.

Children were selected for study who represented a wide range of articulation proficiency and were free of organic deviations related to articulation. Thus, from the pool of some 1500 potential subjects whose articulation had been tested in pre-kindergarten, those with known hearing losses, malformation of the speech mechanism or with known mental retardation were eliminated. This elimination of organic problems was reasonably successful, since at the end of fourth grade only one child had been identified who had a hearing loss of some 35 dB in the speech range, and only 36 of the 450 children remaining in the sample were not in fourth grade. Of these, six were in special classes, 28 were in the third grade and two were in the fifth grade.

To keep the final sample as large as possible, subjects were followed as they transferred to schools within an approximate 25-mile radius of the city. The problem of how far to go to test children never arose since either children moved within the metropolitan area, or they moved so far that it was obvious that they could not be followed. At the beginning of the study, the subjects were enrolled in 45 public elementary schools representing all socio-economic levels in an urban community. By the end of the fourth grade, they were enrolled in 131 schools: 52 city public schools, 47 suburban public schools and 32 parochial or private city and suburban schools. Of the 485 children in the study samples who were tested in pre-kindergarten, 435 remained in the study at the end of fourth grade.

The specific procedures used in a research project must be known and evaluated if the results of the study are to be appropriately interpreted by speech clinicians. The basic data in this study are the perceptions of children's utterances of the phonemes of English. It has been demonstrated that the listener's perception of sounds and the acoustic characteristics of the sounds produced are not necessarily the same (Liberman *et al.,* 1967). Perceptions by carefully selected listeners are deemed appropriate data, since the writer was really concerned with describing the development of articulation in terms of whether or not the sounds of English as uttered are acceptable or unacceptable to those who hear them. However, if this purpose is accepted, then the characteristics of the listeners become particularly important.

The listeners in this study were speech pathologists, most of whom held the Master's degree and had had some experience in the public schools. Thus, they were quite similar in training and experience to the speech clinicians who would likely be the prime consumers of the research findings.

A major problem, however, is that what one person hears is not necessarily what another hears. For many years studies have indicated that listeners agree substantially on the correctness or incorrectness of the production of a phoneme, but that they agree considerably less on how the incorrect utterance is described. Sounds tend to be perceived according to similar features. We can assume, then, that among similarly trained speech clinicians agreement on classification of sounds into phonemic categories is substantial, but somewhat less satisfactory on description of phonetic variations.

Unfortunately, there are no ready techniques to calibrate listeners. In this study, as in most, reliability sessions were held. Agreement among the listeners was quite ·high. However, this is no assurance that the utterances of the children were being accurately perceived. All that can really be said is that every attempt was made to ensure the highest possible agreement of listener judgments for both phonemic and phonetic descriptions. Testers recorded each child's utterances as they heard them. In keeping with the purpose of the study, substitutions of expected phonemes were recorded in broad phonemic transcription, and dis-tortions were described according to phonetic characteristics whenever possible.

The phoneme as uttered in isolated words is the primary, although not the only, articulation unit considered in this study. The phoneme is a basic functional category in speech. It is intimately related to the grapheme used in spelling, reading and writing. Since measures of these language skills are included in the study, the use of the phoneme is essential to provide for the possibility of the widest use of results. The problem of being tied to the status of investigation in a field at the beginning of a longitudinal study has been previously referred to. However, the data in this study have been gathered in a way that concepts such as phonological rules, distinctive features, phonetic environment and the syllable can be used in analyses. In some instances this has already been done.

Children were tested in standard, controlled situations with tests that were selected or constructed for the study. It is a basic premise that the purpose for which any measurement is carried out determines what measure is used. We didn't use the *Templin-Darley Screening Test* or any similar published test in evaluating the articulation of the initial pool of potential subjects because we wished to trace the development of articulation. For this purpose we constructed an articulation test that included all consonants and a number of consonant clusters. Single consonants were evaluated as they initiated and terminated syllables. With the one exception of the / ʒ / in the word *measure,* they also initiated or terminated words. Evaluations were made of all single consonants and of six /r/-, /l/- and /s/-clusters on the longitudinal study samples at each of the test sessions. To explore the relation between shift in accuracy of articulation with and without an aural model and the child's improvement in articulation over time, the same sounds were evaluated in words elicited both by pictures and by the utterance of the examiner.

A number of other measures of articulation were also obtained. Beginning in the spring of the children's kindergarten year, a long articulation test was given at all sessions. It was constructed on the basis of possible linguistic combinations occurring in English words. Imitative utterances of consonants as singles and in clusters were used to evaluate /s/ in 31 items, /l/ in 29 items and various /r/ sounds in 52 items. Other measures of articulation obtained at from one to eight different sessions included the evaluation of sounds as uttered in nonsense words, in sentences, in spontaneous utterances associated with other nonarticulation tests and in a stimulatory measure of words containing the /r/, /l/ and /s/ phonemes.

Administered at selected testing sessions were nonarticulation tests in the speech, reading, spelling, language, auditory stimuli, visual stimuli, personality, intelligence and motor areas. Standardized tests, previously developed research instruments and measures constructed especially for this study were included. The standardized tests included, among others the *Metropolitan Spelling Test,* the *Gates Reading Survey,* the *Wechsler Intelligence Scale for Children* (WISC), *Goodenough Draw-a-Man Test* and the *Bender-Gestalt Test.* Among research instruments previously used were the test devised by Berko to measure understanding of rules of morphological change through their application to nonsense words and the *Templin Sound Discrimination Test* devised to measure sound discrimination ability in identification of minimal pairs of nonsense syllables that were judged as *Same* or *Different.* Several measures devised especially for this tudy were associations of phonemes and graphemes, a dictation spelling test that sampled the understanding of selected spelling rules, attitudes toward speech associated by each child with members of his own family and the pronunciation of unfamiliar words.

Samples with specifically defined articulation characteristics in kindergarten and with articulation that was relatively homogeneous within each sample were provided by the initial classification of the children. These were used for both inter-sample and intra-sample analyses. In the inter-sample analyses, comparisons were made not only of the development of articulation, but also of the relationship between articulation and various other behaviors.

In the intra-sample analyses, attempts have been made to identify factors that might consistently differentiate between subjects with similar articulation at selected test sessions. Within each sample, children have been classified as achievers and nonachievers with second, third or fourth grade articulation test performance taken as the criterion of terminal articulation status. Both articulation and nonarticulation performances have been explored as predictors of articulation achievement at fourth grade. They will be further explored with articulation performance at second, third and eleventh grade taken as terminal status criterion. While a substantial proportion of children with misarticulations in kindergarten can be expected to develop adequate articulation spontaneously, little is known about factors that may identify specific children who will most likely be the achievers or the nonachievers at later grades.

The objective criteria used to classify the children as achievers and nonachievers of satisfactory articulation are somewhat arbitrary. They are test performance criteria which are, in some ways, less desirable than spontaneous speech behavior. However, the criteria were decided upon only after a number of possibilities were explored. One, general intelligibility of speech, was a rating of how well the child was understood by a project examiner. This criterion was used in other work (Templin, 1967) but was not used in this longitudinal study because in it nonachievers were expected to have an articulation deviation sufficient to warrant speech therapy, and children can be easily understood and yet consistently misarticulate one or more phonemes. For example, if a child substitutes the $/\theta/$ for $/s/$, he is still likely to be quite easily understood. Even when a number of misarticulations occur, the correlation between adequacy of production of the phonemes and intelligibility of speech is not necessarily high.

The percentage of children in the elementary grades most frequently reported by speech clinicians as receiving speech therapy has also been used to establish a cutting score for classifying children as achievers and nonachievers in articulation (Templin, 1967). This procedure was discarded when it was discovered that the actual cutting score on the same articulation test varied considerably when the percentage of nonachievers expected was held constant for a number of subsamples drawn randomly from a large number of subjects in the same grade.

The problem of how to define an articulation problem during the developmental period has been faced by a number of persons (e.g. Van Riper, 1969; Wepman, 1967), but no universally accepted criteria are available for classification of children as achievers and nonachievers in the early elementary school years. For this longitudinal study, different criteria of achievement were formulated for the phoneme, shift and percentile samples. For all samples it was demanded that the achievement level necessary for classification as *success* be maintained for two testing sessions, unless the level was reached at the final testing session. In the phoneme samples, to be classified as an achiever it was necessary that the child articulate at least nine-tenths of the 29 to 52 items measuring the production of the phoneme on which he had been initially deficient.

For both percentile and shift samples arbitrary cutting levels were set up for classification of children as achievers or non-achievers. Extensive examination of tests indicated that those whose articulation scores on both consonant single and consonant cluster tests were above 95 per cent of the maximum score could be classified as achievers with confidence. For these no consistent pattern of misarticulations could be identified. Children with scores below 90 per cent of the maximum on both consonant single and cluster tests were classified as nonachievers with reasonable assurance. Examination of their tests indicated that some pattern of misarticulation could be identified. When scores fell between 90 and 95 per cent, however, it was, on the whole, not possible to classify the children as either achievers or nonachievers with confidence. Subjects with scores in this range have not been included in attempts to discover factors that differentiate those who achieve and do not achieve adequate articulation, except in the few instances when they could be classified with confidence.

This longitudinal study must be looked upon as hypothesis-generating. The results that follow do not report all analyses that have been completed, but rather present selected findings that seem to be of particular importance to public school speech clinicians. These findings will later be validated on other longitudinal study data or on independent samples. They are based on analyses of data obtained when the subjects were in preschool through the fourth grade.

The samples selected on the basis of kindergarten articulation indicate that children achieve adequate articulation at widely separated ages. Differences in age are most pronounced among the percentile samples selected according to their number of misarticulations. Adequate articulation was attained by the 98th percentile samples of both sexes by four-and-a-half years of age, by the 50th percentile samples at approximately seven or eight years and by the 30th percentile samples by eight to nine years. However, the 15th and 7th percentile samples had not attained adequate articulation when they were nearly ten years old. At the end of fourth grade the mean scores of the 7th percentile samples approximated those of the 50th percentile samples at pre-kindergarten. On the basis of their articulation scores the relative positions of the percentile samples remained the same either from pre-kindergarten to fourth grade or until about 90 to 95 per cent of the maximum possible articulation score was attained. Thus, for samples as a whole, children who have many misarticulations in pre-kindergarten are likely to continue to have misarticulations into fourth grade.

The shift sample with divergent spontaneous and imitation articulation test scores did not rapidly achieve adequate articulation, as had been expected. The assignment into this sample was based on differences in percentage scores and not on actual shifts to the correct utterance of specific phonemes. The finding, however, has been verified on another sample of 1,000 children in which scores were based on actual shifts (Elliott, 1971). Since the picture and the imitation tests elicit words through perceptual and cognitive channels, it may be that discrepant perceptual and cognitive functions are being tapped. There is also the possibility that these results could be associated with learning disability.

Differences in the rate of development of articulation among phoneme samples were not as pronounced as for the percentile samples. However, the /l/-phoneme sample achieved adequate articulation first, the /r/-phoneme sample next and the /s/-phoneme sample last. Out of approximately 750 possible cases, an /l/-phoneme sample of girls could not be drawn since only five girls were identified who showed the /l/ as a single, consistent misarticulation. The boys' /l/-phoneme sample was smaller than other samples and was made up initially of about 20 subjects, all from about 750 boys who met the criteria for inclusion in it. The /l/-phoneme sample of boys attained adequate articulation at about the same age as the boys' 50th percentile, or normative sample. The /r/-phoneme samples for both sexes reached adequate articulation a few sessions later, and the /s/-phoneme samples for both boys and girls had just about attained it in the spring of fourth grade.

For both boys and girls in the /r/-phoneme samples, the shift from poor to good articulation was frequently saltatory. Subjects shifted from two-thirds or more of the various /r/ sounds being misarticulated to adequately producing all the consonant, vowel or syllabic sounds, /r/, /ɝ/, /ɚ/. The writer had expected that the adequate production of vowel, syllabic and consonant productions of /r/ might be attained at different ages in the same child, but this did not seem to happen. While a similar saltatory pattern was suggested for the boys' /l/-phoneme sample, it is much less firm. For the /s/-phoneme samples the saltatory pattern of improvement was not found.

The relation between articulation and nonarticulation test scores was explored primarily by examining the trends of the 109 mean nonarticulation scores obtained by the several study samples. Since inspection of the scores indicated a tendency to vary with the percentile samples from the 7th to the 98th, the distribution of scores for each nonarticulation variable obtained by each of the percentile samples, boys and girls separately, was classified into one of four categories: (A) Steady increment in mean scores from the 7th to the 98th percentile samples; (B) Saltatory increment in mean scores with that of the 7th percentile sample lowest, those of the middle three percentile samples quite similar and that of the 98th percentile sample highest; (C) Either the 7th or the 98th percentile samples receiving the lowest or highest mean score respectively, with the mean scores for the remaining four samples falling within a relatively narrow range of scores of a different magnitude; and (D) No trend of increase or decrease in mean scores from the 7th to the 98th percentile samples. The first three of these categories indicate a trend toward the 7th percentile receiving the poorer and the 98th the better nonarticulation test scores, but the fourth category indicates no trend.

Approximately 86 per cent of the 109 scores for boys and 94 per cent for girls showed the trend of poorer nonarticulation scores for the 7th percentile samples. The trend was found for both sexes, at all test sessions and on all types of nonarticulation measures. Over 70 per cent of the distributions showed either a steady or a saltatory increase from percentile sample to percentile sample. Differences between the mean scores of the 7th and the 98th percentile samples were significant at the .05 or the .01 level for about 75 per cent of the scores and at the .01 level for about 50 per cent. Specific tests that showed no trend in scores with the percentile samples were administered in various test sessions and included different types of measures: tests in which mean scores were near the maximum (e.g. Murphy-Durrell *Matching Letters)*, those which could be expected to be unrelated to articulation performance (e.g. the *Emotional Scale* of the *Bender Gestalt* test) and some constructed especially for this project.

No clear-cut trend was identified among the phoneme samples. The nonarticulation scores tended to be quite similar, and only in a few scattered instances, were there any differences significant at the .05 level.

The finding that the highest and lowest percentile samples consistently obtained the best and the poorest mean nonarticulation scores over five-and-a-half years after initial testing was not expected. Wepman and Morency, considering many of the same nonarticulation areas, reported no significant differences at first, second or third grade in mean scores of subjects initially selected with acceptable and unacceptable articulation in first grade. The differences between the findings of these two studies cannot be explained by the nonarticulation areas considered, since there is much overlap in these and some in the specific tests used. There are, however, important differences in the characteristics of the samples studies.

Of the completed, more-detailed analyses of relation of articulation to nonarticulation performance, varied degrees of relationship are suggested. One that suggests a strong relationship is that of the application of morphological rules to nonsense words as measured in the test devised by Berko (1958). The child's response was recorded using the International Phonetic Alphabet and classified according to categories such as repetition of the stimulus word, repetition of the stimulus word with the addition of a single consonant, syllable or word, change of stimulus word, etc. A quantitative score, the number of correct inflexions, was also obtained. For this, some arbitrary scoring decisions were made to minimize the effect of misarticulations upon a subject's score for applying morphological rules. For example, the plural of a nonsense word such as *wug,* ending in /g/, a voiced stop, is correctly formed by the addition of /z/, a voiced fricative. Credit was given, not only if the subject said /z/, but if he said any voiced sound, any fricative or any sound he habitually substituted for the /z/. Thus, insofar as was reasonably possible, evaluations of a subject's articulatory and morphological performance were kept independent.

From kindergarten to first and to second grade, the mean morphology scores increased for all samples, but the level of performance of the separate samples differed. For percentile samples, at each grade and for both sexes, quantitative scores increased progressively from the 7th through the 98th percentile samples. Second grade scores of the 7th percentile samples were most similar to those attained in kindergarten by the 98th percentile samples. Thus, there was a two-year difference in the performance of these groups. A 2x3x5 analysis of variance (both sexes, three test sessions and five percentile samples) indicated significant differences at the .001 level of confidence for samples and test sessions, but no significant sex differences. For the phoneme samples, mean morphology scores are not substantially different from one another and probably most frequently resemble those of the 50th percentile, or normative, samples.

The correct application of rules of morphological change seems to follow a pattern similar to that reported by Berko. On the whole, appropriate changes were most frequent when they were achieved by the addition of a sound, next most frequent when they were achieved by the addition of a syllable and finally when achieved by vowel shifts, addition of words or other changes.

A number of factors have been identified in the intra-sample comparisons that may be important for predicting articulation development of individual children. These must, of course, be validated on other samples and are presented here only as tentative findings whose primary value is in suggesting hypotheses for research or therapy.

More analyses have been carried out with the 7th and 15th than with the other percentile samples. A higher proportion of age appropriate misarticulation, as Wepman (1963) has defined them, seems to be a factor identifying children in both the 7th and the 15th percentile samples who are nonachievers at the end of fourth grade. In the 7th percentile samples the difference in the proportion of such sounds misarticulated by achievers and nonachievers reaches the 5 per cent level of confidence beginning with the fall of second grade. In the 15th percentile samples the differences reach this level of significance beginning with the spring of first grade. The 7th percentile sample subjects who did and did not achieve adequate articulation by fourth grade did not differ in kindergarten on the distinctive features they maintained in their misarticulations. A similar analysis is planned, however, at successive testing sessions, and it is expected that the subgroups of achievers and nonachievers may be differentiated at some later sessions. Exploration of the success of basing prediction of spontaneous achievement of adequate articulation upon extrapolation of two consecutive test scores is continuing, since at present evidence is inconclusive.

In the /s/-phoneme samples the possibility of characteristics of the misarticulations of /s/ as predictors of the adequacy of its later articulation has been explored. Similar exploration has not yet been carried out with the percentile samples where children would misarticulate other phonemes. In the /s/-phoneme sample, the most common substitution for the expected /s/ phoneme was the / θ /. About half of the subjects who substituted the / θ / for the /s/ in kindergarten misarticulated the /s/ in fourth grade and about half satisfactorily produced it. This percentage is similar to that reported by Van Riper (1969) for the spontaneous improvement of subjects in his predictive work. No clues have been found that make the / θ / useful in predicting the later articulation of the /s/. However, several characteristics of articulation of the /s/ seem to be predictive. All of the few children who omitted the /s/ (as in *oap* for *soap)* or who substituted a less common sound, such as /t/ for the /s/ (as in *toap* for *soap*) satisfactorily produced the /s/ in fourth grade. Of the children who had produced the lateral /s/ for even a relatively small proportion of the 31 items testing /s/, all seemed to produce an unsatisfactory /s/ in the fourth grade. While these findings were not expected, they can readily be explained in terms either of learning gross rather than fine discriminations or of the amount of overlap in distinctive features between the expected phoneme and the initially substituted sound.

In the upper grades children with substantial deviations are regarded as candidates for speech therapy. This longitudinal study attempts to describe the development of articulation in the early school years and to determine factors that might identify kindergarten children who are potentially deficient in articulation. It attempts to differentiate among children with similar misarticulations those who will slowly develop adequate articulation and those who will continue to misarticulate the phonemes of English and thus to contribute to the formulation of a workable definition of an articulation deviation during the developmental period.

REFERENCES

Berko, J.: The child's learning of English morphology. Word. 14:150-177, 1958.

Bingham, D. S., Van Hattum, R., Faulk, M. E., and Taussig, E.: Program organization and management. J Speech Hear Disord, Monograph Supplement, 8:33-49, 1961.

Bloom, L.: Language Development: Form and Function in Emerging Grammars. Cambridge, M.I.T. Press, 1970.

Blumenthal, A. L.: Language and Psychology. New York, John Wiley and Sons, 1970.

Brown, R., Cazden, C., and Bellugi-Klima, A.: The child's grammar from I to III. In J. Hill (Ed.): Minnesota Symposia on Child Psychology, Minneapolis, University of Minnesota Press, 1969, vol. II.

Chomsky, N.: Syntactic Structures. Gravenhagem, Netherlands, Mouton Press, 1957.

Compton, A. J.: Generative studies of children's phonological disorders. J Speech Hear Disord, 35:315-339, 1970.

Crocker, J. R.: A phonological model of children's articulation competence. J Speech Hear Disord, 34:267-274, 1969.

Darley, F. L., and Winitz, H.: Age of first word: review of research. J Speech Hear Disord, 26:272-290, 1961.

Deese, J.: Psycholinguistics. Boston, Allyn and Bacon, 1970.

Elliott, M. B.: Improvement in articulation with an aural model as a predictor of adequate articulation in second grade. Unpublished paper, 1971.

Friedlander, B. Z.: Receptive language development in infancy. Merrill-Palmer Quarterly, 16:7-51, 1970.

Fry, D. B.: The development of the phonological system in the normal and the deaf child. In F. Smith and G. A. Miller (Eds.): The Genesis of Language: A Psycholinguistic Approach. Cambridge, M.I.T. Press, 1966.

Hull, F., Mielken, P. W., Timmons, R. J., and Willeford, J. A.: The national speech and hearing survey: preliminary results. ASHA. 13:501-509, 1971.

Irwin, O., and Chen, H. P.: Development of speech during infancy: curve of phonemic types. J Exp Psychol, 36:431-436, 1946.

Jakobovitz, L. B., and Miron, M. S. (Eds.): Readings in the Psychology of Language. Englewood Cliffs, Prentice-Hall, 1967.

Jakobson, R. (English translation by A. Keiler): Child Language, Aphasia, and Phonological Universals. The Hague, Mouton Press, 1968.

John, V. P., and Moskovitz, S.: Language acquisition and development in early childhood. In A. H. Marckwardt (Ed.): Linguistics in School Programs. Chicago, University of Chicago Press, 1970.

Jones, H.: Problems of method in longitudinal research. Vita Humana, 1:93-99, 1958.

Lenneberg, E.: Biological Foundations of Language. Cambridge, M.I.T. Press, 1967.

Leopold, W. F.: Patterning in children's language learning. Language Learning, 5:1-14, 1953.

Lewis, M. M.: Infant Speech: A Study of the Beginnings of Language. London, Kegan Paul, 1936, 1951.

Mackie, R. P.: Special Education in the United States: Statistics 1948-1966. New York, Teachers College Press, 1969.

McCarthy, D.: Language development in children. In L. Carmichael (Ed.): Manual of Child Psychology. New York, John Wiley and Sons, 1954.

McNeill, D.: The Acquisition of Language: The Study of Developmental Psycholinguistics. New York, Harper and Row, 1970.

McReynolds, L. V., and Huston, K.: A distinctive feature analysis of children's misarticulations. J Speech Hear Disord, 36:155-166, 1971.

Menyuk, P.: Comparison of grammar of children with functionally deviant and normal speech. J Speech Hear Res, 7:109-121, 1964.

Messer, S.: Implicit phonology in children. J. Verbal Learning Verbal Behavior, 6:609-613, 1967.

Prins, D.: Analysis of correlations among various articulatory deviations. J Speech Hear Res, 5:152-160, 1962.

Pronovost, W.: Case selection in the schools: articulatory disorders. ASHA, 8:179-181, 1966.

Pronovost, W., Wells, C., Gray, D., and Sommers, R.: Public school speech and hearing services, research: current status and needs. J Speech Hear Disord, Monograph Supplement, 8:114-123, 1961.

Shirley, M.: The First Two Years: A Study of Twenty-Five Babies: Intellectual Development. Minneapolis, University of Minnesota Press, 1933.

Shriner, T. H., Holloway, M. S., and Daniloff, R. G.: The relationship between articulatory deficits and syntax in speech defective children. J Speech Hear Res, 12:319-325, 1969.

Siegel, G.: Vocal conditioning in infants. J Speech Hear Disord, 34:3-19, 1969.

Snow, K.: A comparative study of sound substitutions used by "normal" first grade children. Speech Monographs, 31:135-141, 1962.

Snow, K.: A detailed analysis of the articulation responses of "normal" first grade children. J Speech Hear Res, 6:277-290, 1963.

Templin, M. C.: Longitudinal study through the fourth grade of language skills of children with varying speech sound articulation in kindergarten. Unpublished report, Cooperative Research Project No. 2220, U. S. Office of Education, 1968.

Templin, M. C.: Certain Language Skills in Children: Their Development and Interrelationships. Minneapolis, University of Minnesota Press, 1957.

Van Riper, C., and Erickson, R. L.: A predictive screening test. J Speech Hear Disord, 34:214-219, 1969.

Weir, R. H.: Some questions on the child's learning of phonology. In F. Smith and G. A. Miller (Eds.): The Genesis of Language: A Psycholinguistic Approach. Cambridge, M.I.T. Press, 1966.

Wellman, B. L., Case, I. M., Mengert, I. G., and Bradbury, D. E.: Speech Sounds of Young Children. Iowa City, University of Iowa Press, 1936.

Wepman, J. M.: Speech in accuracy in children as related to etiology.

Unpublished report, Cooperative Research Project No. 1198, U. S. Office of Education, 1963.

Wepman, J. M., and Morency, A. S.: School achievement as related to developmental speech inaccuracy. Unpublished report, Cooperative Research Project No. 2225, U. S. Office of Education, 1967.

Williams, F. (Ed.): Language and Poverty. Chicago, Markham Publishing Company, 1970.

CHAPTER IV

VERBAL LEARNING

WILLIAM H. TEDFORD, JR.

VERBAL learning is often confused with two other areas of major concern in psychology: learning theory and linguistics. The first of these is a more general area and is concerned with all types of learning but has traditionally placed most of its emphasis on non-verbal behavior. To the psychologist, linguistics is the study of how verbal associations are assimilated and retained.

This chapter will attempt to survey the field of verbal learning, touching on its major research techniques and findings and pointing up relationships between the work of researchers in verbal learning and in speech pathology. In cognizance of a perpetual problem in clinical speech pathology and drawing on accumulated knowledge from verbal learning research, an approach toward improved diagnostic-predictive methodologies for articulation disorders in suggested at the conclusion of the chapter.

Verbal learning phenomena have been studied systematically for nearly a century. Around 1876 the German psychologist, Hermann Ebbinghaus, was memorizing lists of words and noting those parameters which had an effect on how long he rememberd them. One of the first things he noticed was that linguistic familiarity with material led to easier learning and greater retention. To get around this variable, he invented the *nonsense syllable,* a meaningless but pronounceable word formed by two consonants with a vowel between them. Since there are about 2000 such combinations in the German language, this gave him a large pool of stimuli with which to work. He would write each syllable on a card and then look at each card for a pre-set length of time. He recorded the length of time it took him to memorize a list of syllables and then tested himself, following varying time intervals, as to the completeness of his recall. This led to an observed relationship between amount of material remembered and amount of elapsed time which is still considered valid today; in general, the material turned out to be forgotten very rapidly in the first few hours and more and more gradually thereafter. Ebbinghaus also originated the method of *savings.* He recorded the number of trials taken to re-memorize material he had learned previously; the difference between this figure and the number of trials on original learning could be used as a measure of retention. He also investigated *overlearning,* a procedure in which he continued to review the syllables even after he could recite them without error. Under these conditions the material was forgotten more slowly.

Modern verbal learning experiments have usually used one of three methodologies. *Serial list* learning is very similar to the Ebbinghaus method described above. A subject is presented with a list of words, each of which is exposed to him for a brief period of time. On the second time through the list, the subject attempts to respond with the word following the word which is being exposed. Presentation of the words is usually mechanical, using a memory drum, a device which exposes one word at a time through a small window with the presentation rate being controlled by a motor which rotates the drum. Typical values are a 12-word list with each word being exposed for .5 seconds. The list is repeated over and over until the subject makes a correct recitation, i.e. correctly anticipates each word before it appears in the window.

In serial list learning, each word (except for the first and last) is both a stimulus for the following word and a response to the preceeding word. One method of avoiding this confounding of stimuli and responses is *paired associate* learning. This method employs a series of word pairs with the first member of each pair being a stimulus and the second a response. When the subject sees the stimulus word, he attempts to respond with the associated response word. In this method it is not necessary that the stimulus words be presented in the same order each time, as it is in serial list learning. In fact, the stimulus words are often rearranged after each trial in order to examine the effect this has on learning.

The third methodology is known as *free recall.* The entire list is presented to the subject at one time and then removed. The subject responds verbally or in writing with as many words from the list as he can remember. The interest of the experimenter is in studying the order as well as the amount of recall.

To one not familiar with the verbal learning field, it may seem that restriction to a few methodologies would lead to sterility in research. Consideration of some of the experiments to be described, however, will show that this is not the case. Moreover, there is a great advantage to the psychologist in this voluntary limitation. It means that replication from one laboratory to another is facilitated and that empirical findings can be verified easily. Some of the most "reliable" results in psychology have resulted from studies in verbal learning. Furthermore, these results are beginning to be known and applied in other fields. For example, it has been demonstrated that high anxiety usually facilitates learning of simple tasks but is detrimental to more complex learning, such as distinguishing between sounds which are easily confused. Winitz (1969) has argued that this principle should be applied in articulation therapy so that children with articulation confusions would be corrected only under low anxiety-arousing conditions.

One of the most stable phenomena in verbal learning is the *bowed serial position curve.* Consider a subject learning a list of 12 nonsense syllables, using the serial list method. After the list has been presented several times, he will begin to respond to the first few words and the last few words correctly. As the experiment continues, he makes errors on fewer and fewer words until he goes through a complete trial, or presentation of the list, correctly. If we plot total number of errors for each word on a vertical axis against serial position of the word on a horizontal axis, we usually obtain a smooth curve which peaks just past the midpoint of the list — in this case, around word 7. That is, the subject apparently learns the beginning and the end of the list first, with the middle part being the last to be learned. We can destroy the symmetry of this curve by introducing a *novel stimulus,* or word which is radically different from the others. This might be a polysyllabic word in an otherwise monosyllabic list, or it could be the use of a different typeface or color in printing the word. Novel stimuli which stand out in the list are apparently learned more easily, and the error curve will show a sharp dip at that point. This dip is often called the *Von Restorff effect* after the man who first described the phenomenon.

This leads into the concept of *associations* between words. When word 4 appears in the window of the memory drum, the correct response is, of course, word 5. However, if the subject makes an error, what is that error most likely to be? Many experiments, averaging over large numbers of subjects, have shown that word 6 will be the most likely error. This indicates that the subject not only forms associations between adjacent words but also *remote associations* between words several spaces apart. It has also been shown that these remote associations decrease in strength as the degree of remoteness increases, i.e. word 7 is a less likely response to word 4 than is word 6; word 8 is even less likely, etc. This would seem to have some applicability in teaching speech sounds to children. If the order of presentation of stimuli is always the same, the child may build up remote associations and respond to one stimulus with the sound which is appropriate to the next one on the list. Randomizing the order of presentation could prevent this type of problem from developing.

Another consistent finding has resulted from studies of interference in verbal learning. Suppose we have two groups, an experimental group and a control group, learn a list of words. Call this list A and assume both groups learn it to the same criterion. Then the experimental group learns a similar list, List B, while the control group performs some unrelated task. Finally, we test both groups for their recall of List A. We will find that the control group remembers the list better than the experimental group. This phenomenon is called *retroactive inhibition,* referring to the fact that apparently the effect of learning List B worked backward in time to interfere with material that had already been learned. We can alter the procedure slightly and have the experimental group learn List A while the control group performs some unrelated task. Then we have both groups learn List B and test for retention of List B. Again we find that the control group performs better;

apparently the effect of learning List A works forward in time and interferes with the recall of List B. This is called *proactive inhibition.* The general conclusion that has been drawn from experiments of this sort is that memory is affected by interference from other material, but not by the simple passage of time. Students who wish to maximize recall for examinations are advised to study just before going to bed in order to reduce the amount of retroactive inhibition which would be caused by learning other material immediately after studying. Of course, the longer the time span between learning and recall, the greater the opportunity for interference to occur. This is apparently the reason why the time variable is usually associated with forgetting. Another generality to emerge from these studies is that the greater the similarity between material in the two learning tasks (Lists A and B), the greater the interference. This is somewhat paradoxical, since the greatest similarity would be identity, i.e. the same list would be present both times. However, the latter procedure constitutes a rehearsal trial, or overlearning of the list, and facilitates recall.

Other variables which have been shown to be of importance in verbal learning studies include *meaningfulness* and *intent.* Meaningfulness has been quantified in several ways but a common procedure has been to use the average number of associated words which a group of subjects can think of in a short time period; the greater the number of associations, the greater the meaningfulness of the item. Usually, more meaningful items are learned more readily. Furthermore, paired associate methods have shown that variation in the meaningfulness of the responses has more effect on learning than similar variation in the stimuli. Studies investigating intent have involved letting a subject think that he was an experimental assistant whose task was to read words aloud to another subject. Both subjects can then be tested for recall after having been exposed to the same words the same number of times. Although some learning takes place by the "assistant," it is not as much as that by the subject whose intention is to learn.

Another topic which recently has received a great deal of attention is *short-term memory.* The topics discussed above involve retention over a span of hours or days. Other studies have demonstrated that if the subject is prevented from rehearsing the material immediately after learning it (by interposing some task such as counting numbers backward), a great deal of forgetting seems to occur during the first few seconds. This has led to the concept of two memories: a short-term one in which material can be stored for only very brief periods and a long-term one in which material is placed after being acted upon in some way by the learner.

One difficulty in attempting to survey a broad area such as verbal learning is that one usually concentrates on basic phenomena, and this tends to make the area appear somewhat simplistic. To counteract this faulty appearance, it seems worthwhile to examine a recent and more sophisticated experiment in detail. Tulving (1966) has conducted several studies in an attempt to discover how subjects organize material which they are attempting to learn. His thesis is that material is subjectively organized into what he calls S units. For example, in learning a list of words in which *table* and *chair* occurred, a subject might remember these as a pair, i.e. *table-chair,* where recall of one item would immediately suggest the other. This pair would be an S unit for that particular subject.

Tulving started with two groups of 24 subjects each. Both groups practiced on 18-word lists presented at the rate of one word per second on a memory drum. They were given eight trials using the free recall technique. After these trials, both groups were presented with a new 36-word list and given eight free recall trials. The difference between groups was that the 18 words in the practice list for Group A were included in the 36-word list; the practice list for Group B was not. During the early trials on the 36-word list, Group A remembered more words. However, by trial 5, Group B's recall was superior, and it remained so for the rest of the experiment. Tulving replicated these results using 9-word practice lists and 18-word final lists; they have also been verified by Novinski (1969).

Tulving's explanation is that the organization required for the first list is inappropriate for learning the longer list. That is, the S units learned by Group A help them to recall some of the words, and this is beneficial in early trials while Group B is just getting started. However, Group B builds S units which incorporate the entire list; as they begin to recall over 50 per cent of the words, they gradually surpass Group A. Group A must modify its original S units to eliminate some words and add others. This reorganization interferes with their ability to learn the entire long list as rapidly as Group B.

Tulving had shown earlier that simply reading the words without attempting to remember them had no effect on later learning of the words in a free recall task. Thus, he feels that the subject must organize the words into S units in order to recall very many of them. In other words, the short-memory capacity is limited in the number of items which it can store. This point has been documented rather thoroughly by Miller (1956). In order to recall a large number of words, each *item* in the memory must be a *cluster* of words, or an S unit.

This is a rather sophisticated analysis of learning. It provides some insight into the question of how memory actually operates. It also offers a clue for diagnosis in some types of speech disorders. Consider the case of a child who does not talk, and the associated question of whether the lack of verbalization is due to some physiological factor or to the lack of mental ability. Since most mental ability tests used with children require some form of vocalization, this is often a difficult question to resolve.

Lake and Tedford (1970) repeated Tulving's experiment with the substitution of hand gestures for words. Subjects were shown color slides of a model performing simple hand gestures, such as touching a fist to the chin, placing a palm over the mouth, etc. After each series of slides, the subject repeated as many gestures as he could remember. Otherwise, the procedure was the same as Tulving's. Again, subjects performed better during the early trials of the test list if they had used some of the gestures previously, but on later trials they were out-performed by the group which was naive with respect to the test list. This seems to indicate that subjects organize material of this nature in the same way that they organize verbal material. Further support for this claim is provided by Tedford and Rose (1970). In this experiment, subjects were again presented with slides of hand gestures. One group was provided with verbal labels for the slides and instructed to respond verbally; another group responded by imitating the gestures. Both groups were tested on ability to learn the list using the serial learning paradigm; that is, as each slide appeared on the screen, the subject attempted to respond with the gesture which would be projected next in the series. Analysis of the responses failed to detect any differences between groups in learning rate or technique. Both groups showed bowed serial position curves, improvement over trials at the same rate, etc.

Verbal learning experimenters have accumulated a vast backlog of data on the performance of children with speech defects using motor responses. It should be possible to compare an individual child's learning of a list of gestures to these data. Children whose learning ability is normal could then be distinguised from those who have learning problems in addition to speech defects. A further advantage is that the imitation of gestures should be relatively free of the cultural bias in favor of white, middle-class children which is often found in standard *mental ability* or IQ tests.

Using list learning by imitation to separate children whose learning ability is normal from those whose speech problems are compounded by learning disorders assumes that articulation defects are not due to some underlying motor skills retardation. After a careful review of the literature on this topic, Winitz (1969) concludes that this should be a reasonable assumption.

Van Riper and Irwin (1958) have discussed problems of diagnosis extensively in their chapter on articulation testing and have concluded that there is no test available which will separate those children whose articulation problems will improve spontaneously with maturity from those who require professional help. Many new tests have been devised since the Van Riper and Irwin statement, but the problem still persists. It would seem that research concentrated on the imitative motor ability of children will prove most fruitful in solving this problem.

In summary, it would appear that there should be an overlap of interests between the areas of verbal learning and speech pathology. The methodologies and research techniques which have been worked out in one field may be adaptable to the other. Certainly the large body of information accumulated by psychologists who study verbal behavior should be of interest and of use to the clinician or the researcher interested in the nature of articulation learning.

REFERENCES

Lake, A. E., III, and Tedford, W. H., Jr.: Influence of creativity on formation of subjective units. J Gen Psychol, 83:227-237, 1970.

Miller, G. A.: The magical number seven plus or minus two: Some limits on our capacity for processing information. Psychol Rev, 65:81-97, 1956.

Novinski, L.: Part-whole and whole-part free recall learning. J Verbal Learning Verbal Behavior, 8:152-154, 1969.

Tedford, W. H., Jr., and Rose, Catherine P.: Similarity of verbal and motor learning. Percept Mot Skills, 30:774, 1970.

Tulving, E.: Subjective organization and effects of repetition in multitrial free-recall learning. J Verbal Learning Verbal Behavior, 5:193-197, 1966.

Van Riper, C., and Irwin, J. V.: Voice and Articulation. Englewood Cliffs, Prentice Hall, 1958.

Winitz, H.: Articulatory Acquisition and Behavior. New York City, Appleton-Century-Crofts, 1969.

CHAPTER V

ARTICULATORY ACQUISITION: SOME BEHAVIORAL CONSIDERATIONS

HARRIS WINITZ

MY concerns in this chapter are exclusively with concepts and procedures that may prove to be useful in modifying speech sound behavior, whether of functional or of dialectical origin. The term *speech sound behavior* is a general term that includes phonetic behavior, phonemic status and distributional differences at the phonemic and morphemic levels. No doubt much more than this is involved in speech learning, especially when one considers the new developments in the grammar of phonology. They will not, however, be discussed here.

We shall present below a descriptive outline of three response phases that may have merit for studying phonological learning. Before we do this, we will mention four behavioral processes that are part of each of the response phases. They are as follows:

(1) *Transfer of training.* In psychological theory, transfer is considered to be a general phenomenon that describes or considers a variety of stimulus and response events that influence the learning of a second activity. Given an appropriate set of instances, positive transfer will result. An example of positive transfer at the phonetic level is the following sequence for learning /χ/, a voiceless dorso-uvular fricative:

NOTE: Harris Winitz, "Articulatory Acquisition: Some Behavioral Considerations," *The First Lincolnland Conference on Dialectology,* University of Alabama Press, 1970, pp. 81-96. Copyright by the University of Alabama Press and reproduced by permission.

1. sn*

   ←

2. sn

   ←

   sn

   →

3. h

   ←

   sn

   →

4. /χa/

The principles of this program which are no doubt obvious, result in generalization or transfer of the necessary distinctive features for the utterance of the /χ/ sound. With the exception of this one example I have never devoted my energies to this problem, although it seems worthy of study from theoretical and practical points of view.

(2) *Competition of Responses.* There is little in the psychological literature that will help us understand this problem, although for articulatory learning it is an important dimension. Response competition refers to the blocking or obstruction of new sound learning by highly established responses. These old responses, which by definition are the incorrect responses, may be elicited by a variety of stimuli; for example, distributional cues, morphemic constraints and phonetic and phonemic contexts. The incorrect response may be one or more elements of the phoneme (that is, its distinctive features) or the phoneme itself.

(3) *Auditory Distinctiveness.* It is conceivable that in some instances, speech sound responses may be learned without specialized instruction by using appropriate discrimination pre-training procedures. In our laboratory we have employed the successive discrimination paradigm: it is a two-alternative sound discrimination task. Sounds are presented in random order at five-second intervals and a child attempts to learn which sound

---

*Where sn refers to an inspirated snore and sn to an expirated snore.
   ←   →

corresponds to which of the two buttons or bars.

Difficult sound discriminations can be learned by utilizing the principle of distinctive stimulus pretraining. Learning of difficult discriminations can be effected by utilizing pretraining stimuli that are initially discriminable. In addition, the stimulus elements of the pretraining stimuli and of subsequent stimuli should be from the same stimulus dimension and as similar as possible. Stimulus elements that are both common and similar form the necessary ingredients for mediation and generalization, processes that are no doubt responsible for the effectiveness of pretraining with distinctive stimuli.

The general method is one in which an easy discrimination facilitates learning of a difficult discrimination. No further attempt will be made to give a theoretical accounting of distinctive stimulus pretraining, since it is complex and not very well understood. Its efficacy, however, has been demonstrated with speech sounds in our laboratory (Winitz and Preisler, 1967), using second-graders as subjects. In this study the terminal contrastive pair was /br/–/vr/. The experimental group was pretrained on the /fr/–/br/ contrast, /fre/ vs /bre/, for 48 trials (six blocks of 8 trials). This group received 32 additional trials (four blocks of 8 trials) involving the /br/–/vr/ contrast; the stimuli were /vre/ vs /bre/. The control group received 80 trials (ten blocks of 8 trials) on the /br/–/vr/ contrast (/bre/ vs /vre/). The experimental group benefited substantially from distinctive feature pretraining.

One factor that appears to be a critical component of this procedure is the order of the phonemes used in the training sequence. If the initial contrastive pair includes the correct sound, rather than the error sound, this procedure will not work (Winitz and Preisler, 1967). Presumably, the subject identifies the correct sound as the error sound, or an insignificant variation of the correct sound (allophone in free variation), and the sounds become equivalent during the discrimination session. Thus subjects in our experiment were unable to learn the /ʃ/–/ç/ contrast when /θ/ was paired with /ç/ rather than with /ʃ/ in the early stages of training. It should be mentioned that children most often utter /ʃ/ when they hear /ç/.

(4) *Retention of Articulatory Responses.* A greatly neglected

consideration in articulatory pretraining is the dimension of forgetting. Elsewhere (Winitz, 1969) we have suggested that proactive interference seems to be the most appropriate paradigm for the study of articulatory retention, since older, more established responses are to be replaced by new responses. Presumably the subject brings to the clinic a set of highly learned responses which not only interferes with sound acquisition but affects recall as well. There is an analogue in verbal behavioral research.

Provided with an impressive accumulation of facts, Underwood in 1957 suggested that a good share of the forgetting that occurs in the laboratory may be attributed to events that antedate the laboratory exercise, especially when one observes the cumulative effects of multi-list learning and relearning on retention. Since these antedating associations occur prior to the associations to be recalled and since they are not learned in a laboratory, Underwood and Postman refer to them as extra-experimental sources of interference — associations which the subjects bring to the laboratory and which are detrimental to the retention of new associations learned in the laboratory. The above considerations led Underwood and Postman to consider two sources of interference, letter sequences and unit sequences, that seemed amenable to experimental tests.

In the standard proactive interference (PI) paradigm, two lists are learned in the laboratory; the second list is tested for retention after an interval of time has passed. It can be pictured as follows:

PI Group: Learn A–B   learn A–C . . . . .recall A–C

                        i   k   i   k

Control Group: learn A–C . . . . .recall A–C

                        i   k   i   k

where A refers to stimuli and B and C to responses. A–C recall is superior for the control group, since there is no competition from antedating responses.

When testing for extra-experimental sources of interference, the laboratory exercise involves the learning and retention of a single list. Lists are developed so as to maximize or minimize pre-experimental associations. The associations are assumed to be the result of well-learned natural language habits (NLH) and are gleaned from normative data on associations or computed from their frequency of occurrence in the English language.

The sources of interference in the letter sequence hypothesis are intra-unit and are presumed to operate in the following way. A trigram like *GHO* is relatively infrequent in English. During learning the convert elicitation of frequent trigrams like *GRO* and *GLO* needs to be extinguished. Recall would be difficult because with the passage of time, *GRO* and *GLO* would recover and compete with the recall of *GHO. GRO* and *GLO* would not encounter this kind of competition and therefore should be recalled with little difficulty.

When this theory was originally proposed, no mention was made of the fact that high frequency trigrams may compete among each other to cause a reduction in recall. This consideration has not been tested with single lists, but experiments employing the traditional PI paradigm have not lent weight to this possibility (Postman, 1962; Underwood and Ekstrand, 1967). We are now investigating this situation with single lists in our laboratory.

The unit sequence hypothesis makes opposite predictions for items such as words. High inter-item associations like *square-round, square-circle, square-block, square-box* produce competitive associations maximizing interference and retarding recall. Low frequency words like *lax* or *ado* represent items with a history of few associations, and therefore interference should be minimal. Thus high associations are detrimental for the recall of words but beneficial for the recall of letter sequences. The interference gradients are summarized by Underwood and Postman (1960, pp. 75-76) as follows:

> The letter-sequence interference gradient will be at a maximum when the pre-experimental associative strength between letters is low. The amount of such interference will decrease as the pre-experimental associative connection between letters increases. When the associative connection between letters becomes of strength found among letters in low-frequency words, another gradient, the unit-sequence gradient, begins to emerge. The amount of interference expected from this gradient continues to increase up to the point where very high-frequency words are present.

Over a score of studies aimed at testing the above gradients of interference have given essentially no support to the theory of extra-experimental interference (see Underwood and Ekstrand, 1967). The experimental manipulations have involved a number of verbal behavioral techniques using essentially the list types mentioned above.

SEGMENTATION OF THE ARTICULATORY LEARNING PROCESS

With the above considerations in mind, we have most recently (Winitz and Bellerose, 1968), for experimental purposes, segmented articulatory learning into two major phases of learning: acquisition — learning of a *new* response pattern, and association — linking the newly acquired response to a stimulus.

Using trigrams we can illustrate these two phases most clearly. Thus, for example, learning the following stimulus-response pairs requires presumably first acquisition (or integration) and second association:

Stimulus		*Response*
1	–	XCN
2	–	VGX

XCN and *VGX* are trigrams which do not occur in English. Whereas for the following pairs only association learning is involved:

Stimulus		*Response*
1	–	TOT
2	–	BAB

The grapheme sequences *TOT* and *BAB* appear in words like *total* and *baby*.

An outline of the response acquisition and response association phases is given below.

Response Acquisition

(A) Acquiring sounds that *are not* part of the language.
  1. Some or all features may be available for transfer.

2. Competition is minimal, unless distinctive features overlap considerably.
3. Discrimination pretraining may not be necessary, but possibly may speed up the learning process.
4. Proactive interference is not a factor.

(B) Acquiring sounds that are part of the language.

1. Some or all features may be available for transfer; sounds may be available when the response is inconsistently correct.
2. Competition is maximal, as there is a history of error substitution.
3. Discrimination pretraining may be sufficient if all features are available.
4. Proactive interference impairs recall.

Response Association

1. The sound is available from the response acquisition phase.
2. Competition is from linguistic context and is assumed to be maximal.
3. Discrimination pretraining is effective and may be a sufficient condition for sound learning.
4. Proactive interference impairs recall.

Our own research endeavors have concentrated on discrimination pretraining and retention.

In the brief discussion that follows, we do not refer directly to dialect differences, but perhaps we can make the proper application later in the symposium. No direct mention is made of classical phonemic analysis, since we are often concerned with the learning of a single response. In many ways, however, our outline does take into account phonemic status and distributional differences. The subjects in the studies to be reported were kindergarten, first-, second-, and third-grade children.

RESPONSE ACQUISITION

Acquiring Sounds Not Part of the Language

(1) *Transfer of Features.* In one study (Winitz, 1969) subjects were divided into three groups: (a) perfect articulation (50 correct responses on the Templin-Darley Test), (b) errors of the /r/

phoneme and (c) defective articulation (20 out of 50 on the Templin-Darley Test) including errors of the /r/ and /s/ phonemes. The learning task involved the /vr/ and / ʃm/ clusters. We predicted that on the /vr/ cluster the defective group and the /r/ error group would not differ, and that their scores would be lower than those in the perfect group; and that on the / ʃ m/ cluster, the /r/ error group and the perfect group would not differ, and their scores would be superior to the defective group.

We did not obtain learning for the /vrow/ syllable (20 trials); however, for the / ʃmeɪ / syllable the findings were in the direction stated above. Here, then, is preliminary evidence for response transfer.

(2) *Competition.* We have conducted no study that bears directly on this question, except to say we have taught the phones /ç/, /x/ and /œ/ to children and noted that these sounds can be learned (Winitz and Lawrence, 1961). The order of difficulty from easy to hard was /œ/, /ç/ and /x/. However, for obvious reasons we cannot make any general statements about response difficulty.

(3) *Discrimination Pretraining.* In one study (Winitz and Bellerose, 1967) four subjects (two experimental and two control subjects) learned the /r-w/ and /r̯-w/ contrasts after about three weeks of discrimination training, one-half hour per day. No difference in /r/ production was observed after this extensive period of time.

A phonemic analysis was not made, since all subjects showed no evidence of correct /r/ production. However, had the subjects been inconsistent in their error response and had a phonemic analysis given evidence of an /r/ contrast, we would expect that discrimination pretraining might be sufficient for /r/ transfer. This situation exemplifies response association learning, which will be considered below.

(4) *Retention.* We have no data here, although Rice and Milisen (1954) report that retention was inversely related to the length of the retention interval (one and 72 hours) for teenage subjects. They used the sounds /β/, / ʒ z/ and /x/.

Acquiring Sounds That Are Part of the Language

(1) *Transfer and Competition.* We have no data here, but we

suspect that transfer will be minimal when competition is strong. In short, the rule may be the following:

When the distinctive features of the stimulus compound (the phone) are available to the subject but have a low intrafeature association value, acquisition should be most rapid.

We have by analogy the findings of Underwood and Schulz that trigram learning was inversely correlated (-.78) with an interference index. The index was computed from the single letter transitional probabilities of the second and third letters and the item probability of the first letter. In this instance all letters were, of course, available to the subject, since this was an exercise with the English alphabet.

For sounds, it is difficult to conceive of a situation where distinctive feature availability would not be correlated with some kind of derived distinctive feature associative index. Note in particular that letter associations are linear, whereas for sounds many of the features occur, for the most part, simultaneously. Thus, for the /b/ sound, voicing, stopping and labial movements are for our purposes not a linear association but a *cluster* association. This point of view would not necessarily be a valid one for an acoustical phonetician.

It is possible, however, that the features of voicing, stopping and bilabial placement, for example, may never have been conjoined. That is, consider a child who has no voiced stops and no voiced bilabial sounds. However, he may have a voiceless, bilabial fricative, a voiceless dorso-velar stop and many voiced sounds. In this instance, we would expect that the production of the /b/ sound would take place with minimal interference and maximal transfer.

(2) *Discrimination Pretraining.* Our findings to date do not suggest that discrimination pretraining, when distinct features are available, will result in correct articulatory productions without specialized articulatory training. The evidence we have is extremely limited and is that reported for the /r/ phoneme above.

(3) *Retention.* For the articulatory acquisition stage, retention may be impaired for newly integrated units. The evidence from the verbal behavioral literature suggests that original learning (or interpolated learning in the standard PI paradigm) would be the

critical variable and that, when this was controlled in the studies of extra-experimental sources of interference, the retention of newly integrated units (low frequency trigrams) does not differ from highly integrated units (high frequency trigrams) (Underwood and Ekstrand, 1967).

RESPONSE ASSOCIATION

(1) *Transfer and Competition.* Once a sound has been acquired, positive transfer seems to be related to response competition, the latter being a serious problem in the response association phase. Competition may be from distributional sources; for example, subjects who substitute the /w/ for the /r/ sound in the same environments, say the initial position, would experience response competition. Minimization of the error sound would then be a critical dimension of the response association phase.

In some instances it is possible to minimize competition from distributional sources when the word-unit is a non-English word. The plan here is to integrate the newly acquired sound into word units, sustaining its production over a specified time interval and then gradually transferring it to English words.

Within this general framework, it was hypothesized that the development of an articulatory response would be facilitated when the speech unit does not evoke a previously learned word. It was assumed that the familiar word (mediating response), evoked by a similar verbal stimulus, would elicit an articulatory response to be learned and, thus, interfere with its acquisition. Some support for this hypothesis can be found from the fact that Scott and Milisen (1954) and Carter and Buck (1958) found that the use of nonsense-syllable material facilitated the correction of articulatory errors.

The subjects, first- and second-grade children, assigned initially to one of three groups, were instructed to learn to produce the stimulus /srəb/, which was to be played from a tape recorder (Winitz and Bellerose, 1965). Pretesting had indicated that the majority of children responded to the stimulus /srəb/ with the verbal unit /ʃrəb/. The instructions for the three groups were as follows:

Group I: The subjects were shown a picture of a shrub and were told to learn to pronounce the word shrub in a different way.

Group II: The subjects were instructed to learn to say the *word* they were about to hear.

Group III: The subjects were shown a picture of some cable wires and were told that this was the name of something that goes in a television set and that they were to learn to say its name.

The findings indicate that subjects in Group III benefited from the pretraining instructions. Apparently orientation away from the word *shrub* and to a new *word* reduced the probability that /sr/ and /ʃ r/ would be equated, thereby minimizing the interference of /ʃ r/. Interestingly enough, the word *shrub* did not have to be identified for the subjects, as no difference was found between Groups I and II.

(2) *Discrimination Pretraining.* If orientation to an incorrect perceptual unit retards articulatory learning, then discrimination training should prevent such orientation. Therefore, we decided to test the effects of discrimination training on sound association learning (Winitz and Preisler, 1965).

The subjects were first-grade children, thirty in number, who on two successive days (21 trials per day) did not produce /sr/ when hearing /sr ə'b/. Instead, they uttered /skr ə'b/. (A few children said /ʃ r ə'b/, but the majority in this sample said /skr ə'b/, and so to keep procedures uniform only children with the latter "error" were included.) The instructions they received pertained to the learning situation; that is, they were told to try their best to say the "sound" they heard on the tape recorder and that correct responses would be reinforced.

At the end of the second day, the subjects were divided into two groups: Group A received discrimination training on the /skr ə'b/–/sr ə'b/ contrast while Group B received training on the neutral contrast /sliyp/–/ʃ liyp/. The discrimination procedures were identical to those explained above (under *Auditory Distinctions*).

Discrimination training was conducted on the third day and was continued until ten correct responses in twelve consecutive trials within a maximum number of 208 trials were achieved. The average number of trials for Group A was 72 or about six minutes (the interval of time was five seconds) and for Group B, 44 trials or less than four minutes. Nine subjects, six assigned to Group A and three to Group B, were unable to learn their respective discrimination tasks in 208 trials; they were replaced by new subjects.

The subjects in Group A achieved considerable success; ten of the fifteen subjects responded correctly on several of the posttest trials. Clearly, discrimination training effected correct learning of the /sr/ response.

(3) *Retention.* Perhaps one of the reasons why retention of new articulatory associations is so poor is that there is proactive interference from existing NLH's. Although this hypothesis, as indicated above, has received minimal support from laboratory studies, we made several attempts to test the theory of extra-experimental sources of interference with speech sounds. At least two reasons can be given why speech responses may give positive results where orthographic stimuli and responses have failed. They are as follows: (1) Speech responses should represent the *basic* response level of NLH's, since a written code is usually an inexact representor of a natural language, from which the NLH's are presumed to spring; for example, written word counts may not correspond to spoken word counts, the latter being the assumed source of interference in the above theory. (2) Storage of conflicting responses should follow the oral system rather than the written one; for example, trigram counts that cross syllable boundaries may ill-represent intra-unit associations.

At least one reason can be given for the use of children as subjects in preference to adults. The reason is that given and stated by Keppel (1964, p. 77): "research with children may provide information with regard to new or raw learning, that is, learning which may be considered to have occurred for the first time, rather than being based on previously learned mediators or associations . . . . But these mediators must have been acquired at some time in the history of the subject, and research with children may shed some light on this problem."

The general plan of this study was to teach paired associations involving a consonant substitution, which was designed to elicit response interference. The subjects were elementary school children and were taught a list of four pairs by the anticipation method.

An example of the lists, for the experimental and control groups, is as follows:

List 1 (control group) Stimulus–Response		List 2 (experimental group) Stimulus–Response	
O	vaby	picture*	vaby
X	gog	picture	gog
—	nountain	picture	nountain
∇	shault	picture	shault

*Pictures representing baby, dog, mountain, and salt.

The findings of the several experiments failed to support the assumption that speech sound retention is negatively correlated with associations external to the laboratory situation. Either the design employed here is faulty or the basic theory itself is faulty. However, since PI is a well accepted phenomenon, it seems premature to abandon at this time the concept of extraexperimental interference.

Two segments of the articulatory learning process were considered in this chapter: response acquisition, the learning of new sounds and response association, the integration of sounds within grammatical units, such as words. Behavioral processes presumed to operate in each of these two response phases were discussed under the following four headings: (1) transfer, (2) competition, (3) auditory pretraining and (4) recall.

REFERENCES

Carter, E. T., and Buck, M.: Prognostic testing for functional articulation disorders among children in the first grade. J Speech Hear Disord, 26:124-133, 1953.

Keppel, G.: Retroactive inhibition of serial lists as a function of the presence of positional cues. J Verbal Learning Verbal Behavior, 3:511-517, 1964.

Postman, L.: The temporal course of proactive inhibition for serial lists. J Exp Psychol, 63:361-369, 1962.

Rice, D. B., and Milisen, R.: The influence of increased stimulation upon the production of unfamiliar sounds as a function of time. J Speech Hear

Disord, Monograph Supplement, 4:79-86, 1954.

Scott, D. A., and Milisen, R.: The effectiveness of combined visual-auditory stimulation in improving articulation. J Speech Hear Disord, Monograph Supplement, 4:51-56, 1954.

Underwood, B. J.: Interference and forgetting. Psychol Rev, 64:49-60, 1957.

Underwood, B. J., and Ekstrand, B. R.: Word frequency and accumulative proactive inhibition. J Exp Psychol, 74:193-198, 1967.

Underwood, B. J., and Postman, L.: Extraexperimental sources of interference in forgetting. Psychol Rev, 67:73-95, 1960.

Underwood, B. J., and Schulz, R. W.: Meaningfulness and Verbal Learning. Philadelphia, Lippincott, 1960.

Winitz, H.: Articulatory Acquisition and Behavior. New York, Appleton-Century-Crofts, 1969.

Winitz, H., and Bellerose, B.: Phoneme-cluster learning as a function of instructional method and age. J Verbal Learning Verbal Behavior, 4:98-102, 1965.

Winitz, H.: Relation between sound discrimination and sound learning. J Comm Dis, 1:215-235, 1967.

Winitz, H.: Proactive interference and articulatory retention. Unpublished study, 1968.

Winitz, H., and Lawrence, M.: Children's articulation and sound learning ability. J Speech Hear Res, 4:259-268, 1961.

Winitz, H., and Preisler, L.: Discrimination pretraining and sound learning. Percept Mot Skills, 20:905-916, 1965.

Winitz, H.: Effect of distinctive feature pretraining in phoneme discrimination learning. J Speech Hear Res, 10:315-330, 1967.

CHAPTER VI

PROGRAMMED ARTICULATION THERAPY

EDGAR R. GARRETT

PROGRAMMED articulation therapy is a sub-system of a behavioral modification system of speech and language therapy. When behaviors are approached as performances that can be qualified and quantified, behavioral modification techniques can be applied. The subsequent procedures are quantified, quantifiable procedures can be programmed and programmed procedures can be automated.

A paradigm for planning behavioral modification therapy, long range, session by session and within session, is given in Table I.

In this paradigm, *Entering Behavior* is a description of the subject's articulatory behavior at the time he enters therapy, at the beginning of a given therapy session or the beginning of a particular procedure during a session. Entering behavior is not the

TABLE 1

PARADIGM FOR PLANNING BEHAVIORAL
MODIFICATION THERAPY

Entering Behavior	Terminal Behavior	Methods and Materials	Evaluation

NOTE: The research reported in this chapter was supported by the Arts and Sciences Research Center, New Mexico State University, and by the Bureau of Education for the Handicapped, U.S. Office of Education. Research assistance was provided by Mr. Kay E. Rigg, Assistant Director of the Communication Research Laboratory, New Mexico State University, Mrs. Jean C. Rigg, Programmer and Mr. James A. Boehm, III, Associate Engineer.

same as a traditional diagnosis; entering behavior calls for objective descriptions of behaviors rather than identifying, speculating about or labeling the cause(s) of the behaviors. In planning therapy, there is little value in knowing that a child is lisping because he is imitating a family member, or because he is still using *baby talk,* or because his speech development was delayed because of a long illness. Similarly, there is little value in knowing that on a given articulation test the child lisps in all three positions when the phoneme is single and in the initial position when the phoneme is in a blend. Whatever the case history or articulation inventory may reveal, the clinician still has the responsibility of planning a systematic series of experiences which will modify the child's articulatory behavior so that the child articulates correctly in his on-going speech.

Research with programmed therapy carried out at New Mexico State University indicates that two measures are essential in describing entering articulatory behavior. The first measure is stimulability: given an auditory-visual model of a phoneme, such as /s/, can the child produce the target phoneme in the syllable within three trials; if not, can he produce the cognate, /z/, within three trials? An acceptable production under either condition results in an evaluation of *stimulable* for that phoneme.

The second measure in describing entering articulatory behavior is a *Properant* score. The term *Properant* is derived from the words *proportional* and *operant* and is a measure of the acceptability of the child's articulation in on-going speech (Rigg, 1967). A Properant is made by tape-recording at least a five minute sample of the subject's speech which includes a minimum of 40 attempts at the target phoneme. The clinician then plots the number of acceptable productions of the target phoneme in proportion to the total number of times the phoneme was attempted. A Properant of 1.00 would indicate perfect articulation of the phoneme; a Properant of 0.00 would indicate a total absence of acceptable productions of the phoneme. An actual example of a Properant, with a score of .3, is given in Figure VI-1.

Research at New Mexico State University has shown that the combination of stimulability and Properant score provides a prediction of the probability of change occurring, the degree of

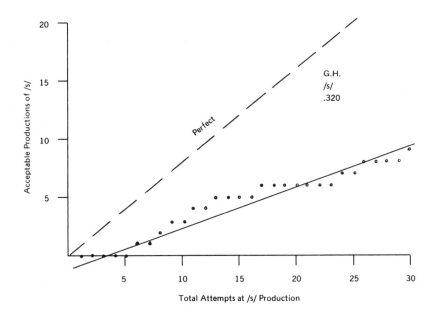

Figure VI-1. Sample articulation properant plot.

change and the time needed under certain programmed articulation therapy procedures. Probability of change, degree of change and time needed will vary according to the type of programmed therapy employed and the type of presentation and contingency employed. Specific examples will be presented later in this chapter. For the moment, the range of articulatory change of a target phoneme for stimulable children is for a mean of .25 on the Properant in 179 minutes with the odds for such a change being eight to one, to a mean of .43 in 23 minutes with the odds being three to one for such a change. When the child is not stimulable, data show that programmed therapy can still be very efficient, but the clinician is not able to predict the time needed, the degree of change nor the probability of that change occurring.

Terminal Behavior in this paradigm is a description of what the subject's articulatory behavior is to be at the termination of therapy. Although the long-range objective is acceptable articulation in on-going speech under everyday normal speaking conditions, terminal behavior is usually written as the behavior desired at the close of a given therapy session; the terminal goal is specified before the session begins.

The type of description recommended is that presented by Mager (1962) in *Preparing Instructional Objectives.* An objective, i.e. the description of the terminal behavior, has three parts: first, a description of the performance or what the subject is to be doing; second, a description of the conditions under which that performance is to take place; and third, the criterion by which the performance is to be judged.

For example, if the decision has been made to use programmed articulation therapy, the first terminal behavior would be concerned with the behavior that is to be present following the presentation of the first script from the self-correction phase of *Automated Stimulus Control System* program, and would read like this:

> Following presentation of the Phase II-1 script for /s/ by the clinician with each correct production being reinforced by a "click" from a counter, the child is to be able to produce /s/ correctly nine out of ten times when the /s/ is presented initially in monosyllabic nonsense syllables, and nine out of ten times when /s/ is presented finally in monosyllabic nonsense syllables. The nonsense syllables will be selected from the script and will be presented at the rate of one stimulus every three seconds. No reinforcement will be provided during the criterion check.

This objective makes it perfectly clear that the criterion of nine out of ten correct productions is expected only when the production conditions and materials are the same as those under which the child had worked; no transfer is expected to conditions with which the child has not worked.

Methods and Materials (the *M&M* Box) is a detailed analysis of the conditions given in the description of the terminal behavior. The sequence which led to the choice of method and material in this example is that the entering behavior of the subject indicated that programmed therapy was appropriate; the terminal behavior was set on the basis of clinical judgement of what could reasonably be expected. In another case the criterion might well have been five out of ten correct; in still another, the criterion could have been ten out of ten. In this example, the entering behavior must have carried an evaluation of *stimulable,* for entry into the ASCS material was made at the first script of the production phase of the program. Since programmed therapy is already available for /s/, no detailed description is needed of the materials. Were materials needed which are not available, this box would contain the details of how the materials were to be prepared and presented.

When programmed materials and methods are used, the requirements of programmed instruction are in effect. A population has been identified and a behavioral terminal goal has been set. The appropriate materials which will lead to that goal are selected, and the material is broken into a multitude of small steps or frames. The usual sequence in programmed instruction is from the *known* to the *unknown.* (The discussion of the ASCS programs which comes later will present one strategy for the preparation of such material.) Since programmed instruction is being used, the method of presentation is also pre-set. Research with the ASCS programs has shown that 2.8 seconds is an optimal frame time to present nonsense syllables to elementary aged children; this period provides adequate time to present the stimulus, have the child respond and provide reinforcement or confirmation. A longer period of time per frame has a detrimental effect upon the child's performance; a shorter period of time per frame is useful only with a few children at this age range.

Evaluation, the last of the four-box paradigm, is concerned with the criterion given in the description of the terminal behavior. In effect, evaluation based upon the stated criterion is an analysis of the adequacy of the projected terminal behavior and/or the methods and materials employed to reach that terminal behavior during the therapy session. The child's achievement of the criterion does not automatically provide a positive evaluation. It is perfectly possible that the criterion was too low and that a higher one should have been set. It is also possible that entry was made at an inappropriate point in the material and that the child was simply demonstrating that he possessed the projected terminal behavior prior to the therapy session. This finding, in turn, indicates that the entering behavior was not properly analyzed.

When the child does not achieve criterion, the clinician should first examine the projected terminal behavior. The degree of correctness specified might well have been too high for the particular stage of therapy. The ASCS research has shown, for example, that some children do not show any significant change in articulation until they reach the sixth script in the production phase of the ASCS.

Method of presentation would also have to be checked if the child did not reach criterion. When the ASCS programs are being used, the clinicians must control the rate of presentation. Clinicians who are not experienced in presenting programmed material tend to let the child set the pace without being aware that the child is controlling the situation. If the time involved in presenting a Phase II-1 script, which contains 50 stimulus frames, exceeded two and a half minutes, the pacing was off, and the clinician's method of presentation was in error.

In the majority of cases, evaluation of programmed therapy will show that the progress made by the child was satisfactory and that the predicted change in articulation is underway.

The examples to this point have centered upon the use of programmed materials that have been previously prepared and field tested. A clinician might well decide to develop materials of his own; in such a case, he should become well acquainted with the literature on programmed instruction in general (Glaser, 1965; Lumsdaine and Glaser, 1960; Skinner, 1953, 1957a, 1957b, 1958, 1960 and 1965) and on programmed articulation therapy specifically (Garrett, 1968; Girardeau and Spradlin, 1970; Holland, 1960; Holland and Matthews, 1963; Sloane and MacAulay, 1968). He should also do some basic reading in behavioral modification and operant conditioning (Bijou and Baer, 1961; Eysenck, 1960; Holland, 1969; Honig, 1966; Krasner and Ullmann, 1965; Ulrich, Stacknik and Mabry, 1966; Wolpe, 1958; Wolpe *et al.*, 1964 and 1966).

AUTOMATED SPEECH CORRECTION PROGRAM

The research at New Mexico State University in the automation of speech and language therapy began in September 1962. The problem was clear: since no change in the number of children and adults in need of and not receiving speech therapy nor in the shortage of certified speech clinicians was predictable, a change in therapeutic procedures was proposed. Programmed instruction and teaching machines had made a marked impact in human learning situations, in many instances being employed in remedial situations where inappropriate responses had to be replaced with appropriate ones. Garrett believed that adequate information and techniques were available for the shaping of acceptable articulatory patterns in cases of functional misarticulation and for the shaping of language patterns, with programmed instruction presented through an automated system.

A. L. Holland (1960) had shown that the discrimination training in articulation therapy for /s/ could be presented as programmed instruction through a teaching machine. She observed an improvement in the articulation of /s/ following training, but the changes were not statistically significant. She also reported that most of her subjects exhibited a spontaneous vocalization of those items composed of words in the successful auditory discrimination training program. These two factors led Garrett to hypothesize that functional misarticulation was amenable to self-correction through programmed instruction.

During 1962-63, an Automated Speech Correction Program (ASCP) teaching machine was designed and built. Programmed instruction was developed for the auditory discrimination and for the self-correction of /s/, /ʃ/, /ɛ/ and /ʊ/. Sixteen college students exhibiting functional misarticulation were used in testing the teaching machine and programmed instruction, with four subjects being assigned to each of the four programs. The subjects completed the auditory discrimination tapes in an average of one hour and ten minutes. The self-correction tapes for vowels were completed in an average of two and one-half hours, and the self-correction tapes for consonants were completed in an average of three and one-half hours. The mean response accuracy on all four programs fell just under 90 percent. Upon completion of the program, each subject could produce the target phoneme on demand, exhibited a marked improvement in his production of that phoneme in test sentences and exhibited some positive degree of transfer of the phoneme to his connected speech. The only therapist aid provided was a brief explanation of an acceptable articulatory posture of the target phoneme between the auditory discrimination and the self-correction phases (Garrett, 1963, 1964).

The first major study in the application of programmed instruction in teaching machines to the automation of speech correction was carried out in the Las Cruces Public Schools in 1964-65. The title of the study was the Automated Speech Correction Program. The major objective was the development, application and evaluation of programmed instruction for the rehabilitation of functional misarticulation of children in the elementary school with the application being made through a completely automated system.

A relatively low-priced teaching machine was developed and tested. A frame time of 6.9 seconds was used, with some nine stimuli being presented each minute. The five ASCP machines proved to be relatively reliable under the extreme demands which were placed upon them. Since a major purpose of this study was an investigation of the effectiveness of different presentation modes of programmed instruction in speech correction, four modes of presentation were available in the ASCP machine.

In the auditory discrimination phase, Phase I of the ASCP, the machines presented the programmed instruction under a *correction* and a *non-correction* mode. Under the correction presentation, a correct response by the subject was reinforced with a 600 cycle pure tone in the earphones, and the teaching machine advanced automatically to the next frame. An incorrect response resulted in the child receiving a *raspberry* or saw-tooth tone in the earphone, and the teaching machine automatically rewound to the beginning of the missed frame and presented it again. Under the non-correction procedure, the subject received a pure tone reinforcer for a correct response, and the teaching machine automatically advanced to the next frame. For an incorrect response, the subject received a saw-tooth tone, and the teaching machine *froze* for a three-second period before proceeding to the next frame.

Two modes of presentation were investigated during the self-correction phase, Phase II of the ASCP. Under the rewind presentation, the subject listened to a master stimulus and recorded his own version; the teaching machine then automatically rewound and presented the master version and the subject's recorded version for his audition. Under the non-rewind treatment, the subject listened to the master stimulus and then heard his production at an amplified level through the earphones as he produced it without a recording being made.

The programmed instruction materials were developed under a Skinnerian straight-line (intrinsic) programming format. A self-organizing system model was introduced, as was the concept of stimulus control programming. The frames of the programmed instruction were so devised that the stimulus for target phoneme was presented in the choices of *Present* or *Not Present, First* or *Second, Neither, Both, First, Second* or *Last, How Many* and *Correctly Articulated* or *Not Correctly Articulated.* The context in which the target phoneme appeared, phonemic, semantic and syntactic, was constantly varied within the 600 frames of the auditory discrimination training program. The order of presentation was determined by establishing an *Ease Index* derived from studies in speech science, information theory, frequency of phoneme and word appearance and frequency and type of articulatory error. The selected criteria were then programmed for an IBM 1620 computer, and the computer-generated syllable and word lists formed the basis of the programmed instruction (Garrett and Rigg, 1964).

A modified randomized blocks design was used with 100 children as subjects; this design allowed an examination of the different combinations of treatment included in the study. One hundred children from the Las Cruces Public Schools were selected with the restrictions that each child be essentially normal in physical condition, emotional adjustment, intelligence, hearing acuity, articulatory structure and be at least seven years, nine months of age but under 12 years of age at the beginning of treatment. The subjects were ranked from high to low according to the summed raw scores of the discrimination and articulation tests used and then assigned randomly, 20 to the control group and 10 to each experimental group.

The positive findings from the study showed that functional misarticulation in normal children between the ages of seven years,

TABLE II

ANALYSIS OF CHANGE IN ARTICULATION
FOLLOWING
PHASE I AND PHASE II TREATMENT
ASCP – LAS CRUCES SCHOOLS

MEASURE	I	II	III	IV	V	VI	VII	VIII
Templin–Darley	<.01	<.001	<.02	<.01	<.01	<.01	NS	<.001
$\bar{\Delta}$ Change: T–D	6.53	5.46	5.86	4.81	6.32	7.93	4.18	8.07

nine months, and 12 years of age could be treated successfully with the Automated Speech Correction Program. The discrimination task in Phase I and the production task in Phase II were apparently well separated insofar as the programmed instruction itself was concerned. No significant statistical difference was found in the performance of the subjects receiving the correction as opposed to the non-correction auditory discrimination treatments. The same finding was true for the self-correction activities under the rewind and the non-rewind presentation. Holland's finding that auditory discrimination on a given phoneme could be achieved in some 20 percent of the time ordinarily allocated in clinical activity was again reaffirmed. Moreover, it had been shown that a generally acceptable, although not stabilized, production of a phoneme could be produced in approximately 20 percent of the time needed under traditional therapy methods (Table III). The general conclusion was that a correction presentation for auditory discrimination combined with a non-rewind presentation for self-correction offered the maximum in clinical usefulness with these particular programs (Garrett, 1965; Garrett and Rigg, 1965).

AUTOMATED STIMULUS CONTROL SYSTEM

The second major study in programmed articulation therapy was carried out during 1965-68 under the title of the Automated

Articulation and Learning

TABLE III

TREATMENT TIME IN MINUTES
ASCS – LAS CRUCES SCHOOLS

TREATMENT	TIME IN MINUTES	
	MEAN	RANGE
Phase I Correction	138	93 to 312
Phase I Non-Correction	98	86 to 121
Phase II Rewind	210	190 to 280
Phase II Non-Rewind	74	- - - - - - - - -

Stimulus Control System. This work was done in four settings; the findings from each setting are presented separately below.

The teaching machines were redesigned so that the subject could respond at any time within a frame regardless of the direction of tape travel and still receive immediate reinforcement. A machanical lock-out device was installed that prevented a subject from pushing more than one button at a time, and a state detection circuit was added which insured that only one pulse would be generated by pushing a response button. The reliability criterion met by the machines before being placed in the field was 2,500 serial frames without a machine failure. Three of the machines in the field were equipped with M&M dispensers and associated logic circuitry, and one was equipped with a synchronized rear screen visual slide projection system. Clinical observation and latency analysis led to shorter frame times of 2 to 3.6 seconds on Phase I and of 6 seconds on Phase II.

The programmed instruction for the Automated Stimulus Control System (ASCS) studies took more than a year to prepare. The Skinnerian straight-line format was retained, as was the basic form provided by the computer-generated word lists. An error analysis of the original ASCP programmed instruction was made, and the identifiable error sources were eliminated with far more rigid control being exercised in the introduction of contrasting phonemes, the influence of adjacent phonetic elements, the effect of frequency of use and familiarity, the semantic influence of word choice and the *depth* of the syntactic material. The stimulus control element in the programs was strengthened, and a backward chaining sequence was introduced in the production phase of the programs. *Button-Training Tapes* were written to teach the button-pushing task to the subjects prior to their work with the programs proper, and the instructional sections or *Training Tape Leaders* were rewritten and expanded.

At the Dixon State School, Dixon, Illinois, the major objective was a study of the application and evaluation of programmed instruction for the correction of functional misarticulations in educable mentally retarded children. The experimental design allowed for the comparison of the relative effectiveness of programmed instruction and teaching machines with one experimental group receiving a pure tone reinforcer and the second experimental group receiving the pure tone reinforcer together with a randomized fixed-ratio M&M reinforcer set at 40 percent. A third group of subjects received traditional therapy from certified speech clinicians.

Thirty-two mentally retarded patients with functional misarticulation problems were selected as subjects. All subjects were in normal physical condition, without severe emotional maladjustment, ranked in the 50 − 75 I.Q. range, had normal auditory acuity, possessed normal structural relationships of the articulatory organs and essentially normal movement, showed misarticulation of at least two General American phonemes and were between 8 and 16 years of age.

The effect of the ASCS treatment on the articulation of educable mentally retarded subjects is shown in Table IV.

The ASCS programs were effective when only the pure tone was used as a reinforcer. The ASCS programs were not effective when pure tone plus M&M were used for reinforcement. Reports from Dixon indicated that the M&M dispenser served as a distraction to the learning task, and this impression was confirmed by examination of the latency and error rate of subjects receiving this treatment. Another important finding was that the subjects who

TABLE IV

ANALYSIS OF CHANGE IN ARTICULATION
FOLLOWING
PHASE I AND PHASE II TREATMENT
ASCS – DIXON STATE SCHOOL

MEASURE	TREATMENT	MEAN DIFF.	S.E. DIFF.	t	P
Templin-Darley Articulation	M&M and Tone Reinforced	5.08	3.63	1.46	NS
	Tone Only Reinforced	4.98	2.07	2.50	< .05
	Traditional Therapy	10.95	4.78	2.10	NS

received traditional therapy did not show a significant change in articulation although their mean change on the Templin-Darley test was greater than that of the subjects receiving the ASCS treatment. Also, the total time involved in traditional therapy was greater than that for the ASCS treatments.

At the Atlanta Speech School, Incorporated, Atlanta, Georgia, the major objective was a study to determine whether children with aphasia (language disorders) would profit from automated instruction with respect to articulatory skill and show improvement in rate and accuracy of response after auditory discrimination training. The study was designed so that a comparison could be made of the relative effectiveness of the Automated Stimulus Control System on aphasic children with normal hearing as opposed to aphasic children with questionable hearing. Reinforcement for both groups was provided by the combination of pure tone and M&M dispenser, with the latter set for 60 percent.

Twenty subjects were selected from the 46 children enrolled at the Atlanta Speech School, Incorporated. The subjects ranged in age from 4 to 14 years. Half had normal hearing, and half had auditory acuity that was less clearly defined and for whom there was a possibility of moderate reduction in acuity. Standard performance type tests indicated an I.Q. range of 81 to 131, with a mean of 102 and median of 101.

The results from the studies at the Atlanta Speech School are incomplete, but the analysis is sufficiently interesting to be reported. One subject was eliminated from the study, and complete data are available on only nine of the 19 remaining subjects. The nine subjects include both children with normal hearing and those with questionable hearing. The positive results experienced by these children is given in Table V.

At the Veterans Administration Speech Pathology and Hearing Service, Atlanta, Georgia, the major objective was an exploratory study to determine whether adults diagnosed variously as oral apractics, peripheral dysarthriacs or aphasics would profit from automated instruction of the type offered by the ASC System. The limited and unpredictable number of subjects available for the study prohibited an experimental design. Six Veterans Administration out-patients and one in-patient who were diagnosed variously as having mild to severe aphasic symptoms were the subjects. The auditory discrimination phase of the treatment was completed by three subjects. The self-correction phase was not used with any subject. No clinical change in speech or language behavior was

TABLE V

ANALYSIS OF CHANGE IN ARTICULATION
FOLLOWING
PHASE I AND PHASE II TREATMENT
ASCS – ATLANTA SPEECH SCHOOL, INC.

MEASURE	*TREATMENT*	*MEAN DIFF.*	*S.E. DIFF.*	t	*P*
Templin-Darley Articulation	M&M and Tone Reinforced	7.89	2.00	3.95	.01

observed for any of the patients. An analysis of the responses of
the patients who completed the Phase I treatment indicated that
their responses were not random, but the pattern of responses
could not be identified.

At the Las Cruces, New Mexico, schools the objectives were (1)
a clinical evaluation of the effectiveness of the ASC System when
the teaching machines were placed in public school settings and
administered solely by non-professional school personnel and (2) a
clinical evaluation of the effectiveness of the programmed instruction when it was presented by a speech clinician to groups of
children. This clinical evaluation did not require an experimental
design, but a design comparing presentation by machine to
presentation by clinician was evolved to provide more information
about the effectiveness of the programmed instruction materials.
The machines used in the Las Cruces schools were the original
ASCP teaching machines; the programs were the revised ASCS
programmed instruction.

Three elementary schools in the Las Cruces system each
provided 20 subjects. One group of ten subjects at each school
received the ASCS programmed instruction on teaching machines
under regular school personnel. The other group of ten subjects at
each school received the ASCS programmed instruction in groups
of two to four children from a certified speech clinician.

The positive results in articulatory change produced by both
treatments are shown in Table VI.

One major finding from this study was that programmed
instruction presented by teaching machine without the supervision
of a certified speech clinician could produce a positive change in
the articulatory pattern of children with functional misarticulation. The second major finding was that a speech clinician could
present the programmed instruction to groups of four children as
efficiently as the teaching machine presents the same material to
an individual child. Because of the clinical nature of the study in
the Las Cruces Schools, no record was kept of time. Since the
machine subjects in this setting were working on the original ASCP
machines, a safe estimate is that they averaged approximately 130
minutes on Phase I and 50 minutes on Phase II. The time for the
clinician-presented ASCS treatment was markedly less; she was

TABLE VI

ANALYSIS OF CHANGE IN ARTICULATION
FOLLOWING
PHASE I AND PHASE II TREATMENT
ASCS–LAS CRUCES SCHOOLS

MEASURE	TREATMENT	MEAN DIFF.	S.E. DIFF.	t	P
Templin-Darley	Machine Administered	8.24	1.67	4.94	$< .001$
Articulation	Clinician Administered	8.31	1.95	4.19	$< .001$

working with groups, and she averaged a frame time of four seconds throughout the program as opposed to the 6.9 seconds frame time of the machine.

An extremely interesting finding was that all of the subjects, the retarded children, the aphasic children and the aphasic adults, varied though they took essentially the same time to complete the programs, as shown in Table VII.

Standard procedures had been followed in the ASCP and ASCS studies that required each subject to go through both the discrimination and production phases of the program, with the changes being measured by an articulation test (Templin and Darley, 1960) and a discrimination test (Templin, 1943). Several puzzling anomalies emerged together with the positive finding that an automated program was effective.

The first anomaly was the regression in discrimination as measured by the discrimination test from a significant level immediately following completion of the discrimination training to a non-significant level following the self-correction training. A time-honored belief held that discrimination was needed if production were to change, but the ASCP and ASCS data did not support that assumption.

TABLE VII

ASCS TREATMENT TIME IN MINUTES

SETTING	TREATMENT	RANGE PHASE I	MEAN PHASE I	PHASE II	MEAN TOTAL
Dixon State School	ASCS Tone Reinforced	140-521	253	53	306
	ASCS M&M Reinforced	159-346	228	53	281
	Tradition Therapy	N/A	N/A	N/A	356
Atlanta Speech School	ASCS M&M Reinforced	231-292	262	53	315
Atlanta V.A.	ASCS Tone Only Reinforced	200-290	230	–	–

The second anomaly was the apparent contradiction that lay between the positive change in articulatory behavior and the high error rate shown on the programmed instruction. For example, the normal children had shown a mean error rate on Phase I of the program, which dealt with discrimination training, of 23.3 per cent in a range of 1.1 to 125.0 per cent (it was possible to respond more than once to each frame under the correction mode). The error rate in Phase II of the program, which provided for production under self-correction conditions, had been equally high. The philosophy in programmed instruction at the time was that an error rate in excess of 10 per cent was the mark of an ineffectual program. This was obviously not the case.

Exploratory studies with the Properant and stimulability

TABLE VIII

ANALYSIS OF CHANGE IN TEMPLIN-DARLEY
FOLLOWING
PHASE I AND PHASE II TREATMENT
ASCS–LAS CRUCES SCHOOLS

SUBJECTS (N = 50)	MEAN DIFF.	t	P
Total	7.66	5.98	< .001
Stimulable	8.75	4.35	< .001
Non-Stimulable	6.65	4.06	< .001

measures had been completed when the ASCS study in the Las Cruces Schools was initiated, so Properant and stimulability measures were included with the standard measures and appropriate analyses were made.

Since both the machine and clinician treatment had been the complete ASCS program under the same conditions of reinforcement, the data for 50 subjects who completed the treatment were lumped. As Table VIII shows, when articulatory change as measured by the Templin-Darley was examined, the factor of stimulability provided no information beyond that already found (Table VI).

However, when articulatory change as measured by Properant score was examined, stimulability became the major factor, as shown in Table IX.

These analyses led to certain conclusions concerning the use of ASCS programmed therapy. First, the need, indeed the value, of putting a stimulable child through the discrimination phase of the program is extremely suspect; stimulables have a production available, and the focus should be directed toward increasing the rate of and the generalization of the production. Second, change in articulatory behavior as measured by the Templin-Darley does not correlate to the actual change in on-going speech as measured

TABLE IX

ANALYSIS OF CHANGE IN PROPERANT
FOLLOWING
PHASE I AND PHASE II TREATMENT
ASCS–LAS CRUCES SCHOOLS

SUBJECTS (N - 50)	MEAN DIFF.	t	P
Total	.153	4.72	<.001
Stimulable	.255	6.00	<.001
Non-Stimulable	.059	1.44	N. S.

by the Properant. Since change in on-going speech is the ultimate goal of the clinician, the Properant is the more appropriate measure. And third, it is possible to predict the degree of change in Properant score for stimulables; treatment with the ASCS under the conditions of this study will produce a Properant gain of at least .15 with the probability of success being .9.

MICROUNITS

McLean's research in the use of operant techniques to extend stimulus control of phoneme articulation (McLean 1965a, 1965b, 1967, 1970; McLean and Spradlin, 1967) represents another type of programmed therapy developed under a learning theory paradigm. The research was carried out at the Parsons State Hospital and Training Center, Parsons, Kansas, with institutionalized male residents. McLean's general plan was to establish a specific procedure of programmed antecedent stimulus conditions under positive reinforcement contingencies. His specific plan was, first, to evoke the target phoneme in words by presenting echoic stimuli for the subjects to imitate and subsequently to shift the correct response to the control of three types of stimuli which had

TABLE X

SAMPLE PROGRAM FOR INITIAL /s/

Stimulus Conditions

	S Echoic	S Picture	S Grapheme	S Intra-verbal	S S S Functional
Sew					
Sock					
Sip					
Seat					
Saddle					

(+) = Correct Articulation of /s/

(–) = Incorrect Articulation of /s/

not previously evoked the correct response. These three types of stimuli were pictures, graphemes of the words and intraverbal chains. Table X shows a sample program for /s/.

Each program consisted of ten words. The words were presented under the echoic (s^1) condition until the subject reached criterion of 50 per cent correct on four successive blocks. A picture stimulus (S^2) was then paired with the echoic stimulus by the clinician holding the picture close to his mouth as the word was spoken. When the subject reached criterion of 20 correct responses in 20 paired presentations, the echoic stimulus was withdrawn, and the response was evoked by the picture stimulus alone. Criterion with the picture stimulus was 38 correct productions out of 40 presentations. The same pairing between conditions and the same criterion of 38 out of 40 applied to the grapheme (S^3) and intraverbal (S^4) conditions.

McLean has found that this type of programmed therapy changed phoneme articulation in words under the four stimulus conditions with high efficiency, that the learned phoneme generalized to untrained words in the great majority of subjects, that the majority of subjects tended to overgeneralize the learned phoneme to their old substitution phonemes and that none of the mentally retarded subjects generalized the learned phoneme to a new position. Subsequent practice was needed for the phoneme to transfer into connected speech, as indicated by the *Functional Condition* in Table X.

This program was usually completed after the presentation of 78 training blocks of ten items over a two-and-a-half week period. The program has been so successful that McLean is now concentrating upon the development of responses which are not easily attained by imitative procedures (McLean, 1969).

Garrett modified McLean's procedure for several studies carried out with normal public school children. The criterion for passing from one training condition to the next was reduced to ten out of ten successive correct productions; the pairing of conditions was dropped; a maximum of three seconds was set for the presentation of the stimulus, the response and the reinforcement under the echoic, pictoral, graphemic and interverbal conditions; and the functional (S^5) condition was included as a regular part of the treatment. The term *Microunit* was applied to the modified procedure.

Two experienced public school clinicians were trained in the use of Microunits, and ten randomly selected cases received the treatment in an exploratory study. Three cases with lateral or fronted /s/ were corrected in an average of 60 minutes of therapy; one case with a /w-1/ substitution was corrected in 45 minutes; two cases with /r/ distortion were corrected in 18 and 8 minutes, respectively; and four cases with /ʃ/ distortion or /ʃ-tʃ/ confusion showed significant improvement after 30 minutes of therapy.

The findings from this exploratory study confirmed McLean's report that phoneme articulation in words changed with high efficiency under the first four stimulus conditions and that the learned phoneme generalized to untrained words in all subjects. But unlike the retardates who were the subjects in McLean's study, these ten normal children did not over-generalize the learned phoneme to their old substitution phoneme, and all of the subjects generalized the learned phoneme to a new position, although not all subjects did so consistently.

Following the exploratory study with Microunits, the same two clinicians carried out a major study of programmed articulation therapy in the El Paso, Texas, public schools. One portion of the study was concerned with Microunit therapy and involved 41 subjects. These subjects showed a mean positive change of .42 on their Properant scores after an average of 23 minutes of individual therapy. All 41 subjects achieved criterion under the echoic, pictorial, graphemic and interverbal conditions; all 41 subjects generalized production of their target phoneme to untrained words; and 36 subjects generalized the target phoneme to other positions. Five subjects did not generalize their target phoneme to other positions, did over-generalize to their previous substitution phoneme and needed a paired presentation in order to progress from one training condition to the next. In effect, these five children exhibited the type of behavior reported for McLean's retardates.

PROGRAMMED ARTICULATION THERAPY IN AN ON-GOING PROGRAM

The study in the El Paso, Texas, schools provided an opportunity to examine the relative effectiveness of the ASCS program and Microunits in changing the articulatory behavior of school children in an on-going school therapy program. The director of special education in the system granted permission for the clinicians to shift from group to individual therapy, to employ programmed materials in their therapy and to carry out the study.

To avoid scheduling changes, the clinicians continued to have groups of children report as usual, but all articulation therapy was carried out individually with each child receiving from five to seven minutes of individual attention at each of the two weekly sessions. No problems arose with the children who were not actively involved; they were permitted to return to their classrooms after they had completed their scheduled program, or to stay in the speech therapy room and read or otherwise occupy themselves. During the last month of therapy, a number of the children became actively involved in the therapy process and presented microunits to other children. Each clinician carried a case load of 100. A total of 152 children received programmed articulation therapy; the remaining 48 cases had other problems.

By the end of February, 1969, when the study was initiated, all of the children had been in therapy for a number of months; a number had been receiving therapy for more than a year. A Properant was taken during the first week of March as the pre-treatment measure; a second Properant was taken during the third week of May as the post-treatment measure. All of the children were *stimulable* in that they could produce the target phoneme, or its cognate, in a nonsense syllable when the phoneme was modeled by the clinician. Since all of the children were stimulable, all discrimination training was stopped and the ASCS Phase II or production programs and the Microunits were specified as the treatments. The clinicians assigned the children to the ASCS or Microunit treatment on an essentially random and definitely arbitrary basis. A finger-press counter which emitted a loud "click" was used both to provide reinforcement and to record the number of correct responses during a session. Detailed records were kept for each child and included information on the number of attempted productions, the number and identity of accepted and reinforced productions and the time actually spent during each individual therapy period.

Of the 152 articulation cases, 74 received only Phase II ASCS programs, 41 received only Microunits and 37 received a mixture of ASCS and Microunits. The clinical judgment of the two clinicians provided the impetus for the mixed treatments, judgment that was supported by the positive gains made by the 37 subjects. However, no specific pattern had been followed in shifting from one treatment to the other, so the data from the mixed treatment subjects could not be included in the statistical analysis.

As indicated in Table XI, the mean time in therapy was 26 minutes for the ASCS subjects and 23 minutes for the Microunit subjects. The quite different range of time for the two treatments is important and will be discussed later.

The mean gain in articulation of the target phoneme as

TABLE XI

TREATMENT TIME IN MINUTES
EL PASO SCHOOLS

| TREATMENT | TIME IN MINUTES | |
	MEAN	RANGE
Microunits	23	9 – 64
ASCS	26	16 – 36

TABLE XII

ANALYSIS OF CHANGE IN ARTICULATION
EL PASO SCHOOLS

MEASURE	TREATMENT	RANGE	MEAN CHANGE	t	df	P
Properant	Microunits	.04 – .81	.42	5.78	39	<.001
	ASCS	.03 – .66	.34	7.68	72	<.001

measured by change in the Properant score, as shown in Table XII, was .34 under the ASCS treatment and .42 under the Microunit treatment. Again, the range of change under the two treatments is important and the implications will be pointed out.

DECISION MODEL FOR PROGRAMMED ARTICULATION THERAPY

Further consideration of the data available from the El Paso schools study of programmed articulation therapy led to a graphic

analysis of the change in Properant against the time in individual
therapy to produce that change. The plot is given in Figure VI-2.
The most notable feature about Figure VI-2 is that the larger
Properant changes are associated with the short times required to
complete treatment for both the ASCS programs and the
Microunits.

By smoothing the curves in Figure VI-2, the cost-effectiveness of
the two types of programmed therapy used in the study become
apparent (Figure VI-3). The cost-effectiveness curve becomes

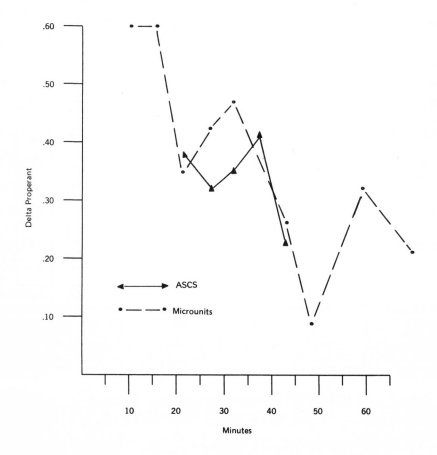

Figure VI-2. Change in properant versus time in training.

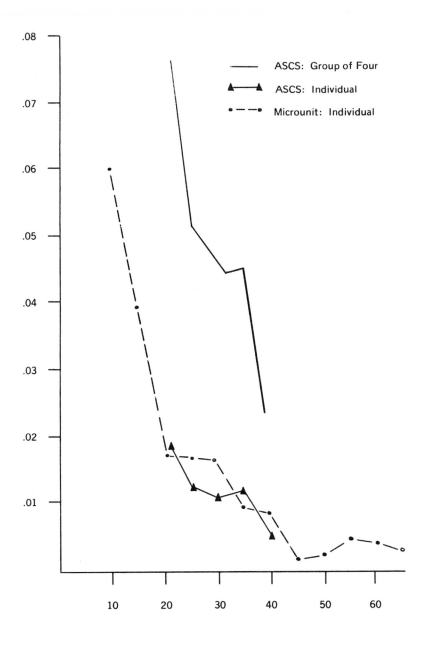

Figure VI-3. Cost effectiveness versus time.

asymptotic with zero at about 60 minutes; in other words, the greater the amount of time needed to produce change, the less change that is produced per minute of therapy. Restating again, the amount of time spent on both the Microunit and the ASCS is inversely related to the change in articulatory behavior as measured by the Properant.

Further consideration of the data showed that the amount of time necessary to reach criterion in the echoic condition of the Microunit is highly correlated with the amount of time necessary to complete the other four conditions of the Microunit (Kendall rank coefficient is .81, with $p < .001$).

These two pieces of information led to asking what cut-off time for the echoic portion of the Microunit would optimize the power of the Microunits while at the same time allowing the shift of slow responders to the ASCS where they should make a greater change than if left on the Microunit treatment. Three and a half minutes is the answer. Using the three and a half minute criterion, records showed that the subjects meeting this criterion had a mean Properant change of .477, whereas those who would have been rejected had a mean Properant change of .341. Had these subjects been shifted to ASCS when they failed to meet the three and a half minute criterion on the echoic portion of the Microunit, their predicted mean Properant would have been .380 with a significant saving in time.

The El Paso data confirmed previous findings about the ASCS program and supported the hypothesis about the predictive value of stimulability and the utility of the Properant. With stimulable children receiving the production phase of the ASCS program under a constant schedule of reinforcement for correct productions, the minimum prediction is a Properant increase of .250 with a probability of success of .9. With stimulable children receiving the Microunit treatment after meeting the three and a half minute criterion on the echoic portion, the minimum prediction is a Properant increase of .300 with a probability of success of .6.

These findings resulted in a decision model for clinicians to follow in using programmed therapy with stimulable children. The model is presented in Figure VI-4.

The one additional bit of information in the model is the

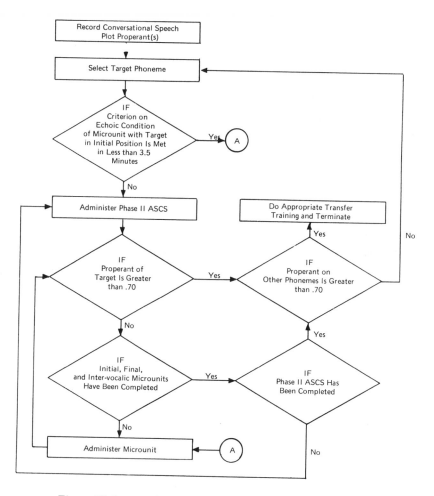

Figure VI-4. Decision model for stimulable children.

Properant of .70 as the exit point from the programmed therapy. The cost-effectiveness analysis showed clearly that little change would result from additional therapy after the first 60 minutes. Of equal importance was a study of retention of articulatory change in the target phoneme two weeks after termination of therapy: 90 per cent of the El Paso subjects who had received a .70 Properant were maintaining or exceeding their post-treatment Properant. The conclusion was that a child with performance at the .70 level found ample reinforcement for good articulation in his on-going environment; the clinician had brought the child to the point where the contingencies in the on-going communication process were in control.

This decision model does not cover all the cases in need of articulation therapy. Research underway with programmed articulation therapy at New Mexico State University and elsewhere should soon produce models and procedures that will enable the practicing clinician to deal with the stimulable child who does not respond to the ASCS or Microunit treatment and with the non-stimulable child whose performance cannot now be predicted. It should be clearly understood that non-stimulable children frequently show marked improvement under both the ASCS and Microunit treatments. Some of the greatest individual changes made in these studies were made by non-stimulable children. The difficulty is that no measure is yet available which will predict what change in articulatory behavior can be achieved in a given period of time with such children.

IMPLICATIONS

The implications from these studies fall into two major groups. The first set of implications has to do with automated therapy; the second has to do with clinician-presented programmed therapy.

The studies of the Automated Stimulus Control System produced three important implications. The first is that the public school clinician could handle the majority of his functional misarticulation cases with an automated system. This implication is valid even though it is evident that the clinician is reluctant to adopt a machine system for a task which he has been taught can be handled only through the direct interaction of clinician and student. Until the clinician sheds this reluctance, he will not press his administrators for teaching machines; and his administrators are not likely to press him.

The second implication is that the availability of an automated system would enable schools without clinicians to provide speech correction services by utilizing the system through non-professionals. The resistance to change in school programs of all types works against the adoption of such a system. After years of positive reports from research studies, only a few scattered instances can be found of classroom instruction being carried out solely by teaching machine or computor, to say nothing of programmed instruction in other forms. It is safe, unfortunately, to assume that a fairly long period will pass before automated speech therapy is available in settings without speech clinicians.

The third implication is that an automated system of programmed therapy would be especially valuable for mentally retarded and language disabled individuals whose speech needs can be met only through long periods of therapy. An automated system would provide an optimal learning situation in a format which would allow for the repetitive and patient procedures needed by these individuals. Unfortunately, the probability of change in special education settings is not much higher than the probability in regular education settings.

The implications coming from clinician-presented programmed therapy carry the greatest promise for change in public school therapy in the immediate future. Of these implications, two stand out. The first is that the clinician can make predictions about the performance of the children with whom he works. Two predictors are available: stimulability, which enables him to predict that a given child will respond positively to programmed therapy and the echoic condition of the Microunit, which enables him to predict which treatment will produce the greatest change in the child's performance.

The second implication is that the clinician can justify his procedures in terms of dollars and cents. The cost-effectiveness analysis of programmed therapy places a major part of the typical school therapy program on a financial justification level not yet available to most school programs.

IMPLEMENTATION

Implementation of programmed articulation therapy, and of behavioral modification therapy in general, rests with the school clinician. Before such procedures are adopted, he must accept the evidence that shows that efficient methods for controlling human behavior are available, and he must make the ethical decision to use these methods. Once these steps are taken, the clinician will change from artist to scientist. The hallmark of science is the ability to predict; programmed articulation therapy does enable the clinician to make reliable predictions.

The decision to use programmed therapy is worthless unless the clinician modifies his own behavior. He must shift to individualized therapy, schedule brief periods of intensive therapy, increase his rate of stimulus presentation and reinforce the high rate of response on the child's part. The most difficult task for the clinician will be to adhere to programmed therapy procedures when his subjective reaction interferes. He can make that step if he is willing to manipulate his own contingencies; the reward in programmed therapy comes with the change in the child's performance, not from the clinician's own feeling of security.

REFERENCES

Bijou, S. W., and Baer, D. M.: Child Development: A Systematic and Empirical Theory. New York, Appleton-Century-Crofts, 1961.

Eysenck, H. J.: Behavior Therapy and the Neuroses. New York, Pergamon Press, 1960.

Garrett, E. R.: An automated speech correction program: a pilot study. Paper read at American Speech and Hearing Association 1963 National Convention. Abstracted in Asha, 5:796, 1963.

Garrett, E. R.: Correction of Functional Misarticulation under an Automated Self-Correction System: Summary Report. Submitted to the U. S. Office of Education, Project Number 2749, 1965.

Garrett, E. R.: Scientific exhibit award winner: an automated speech correction program. Asha, 6:87, 1964.

Garrett, E. R.: Speech and Language Therapy under an Automated Stimulus Control System: Final Report. Submitted to the U. S. Office of Education, Project Number 3192, 1968.

Garrett, E. R., and Rigg, K. E.: Automated self-correction of functional misarticulation in the public schools. Paper read at the American Speech and Hearing Association 1965 National Convention. Abstracted in Asha, 7:422, 1965.

Garrett, E. R., and Rigg, K. E.: Computer-generated word lists for articulatory improvement. Paper read at the American Speech and Hearing Association 1964 National Convention. Abstracted in Asha, 6:393, 1964.

Girardeau, F. L., and Spradlin, J. E. (Eds.): A functional analysis approach to speech and language. ASHA Monographs Number 14 (1970).

Glaser, R. (Ed.): Teaching Machines and Programmed Learning, II. Washington, D. C., Department of Audiovisual Instruction, National Education Association of the United States, 1965.

Holland, A. L.: The Development and Evaluation of Teaching Machine Procedures for Increasing Auditory Discrimination Skill in Children with Articulatory Disorders. Unpublished doctoral dissertation, University of Pittsburgh, 1960.

Holland, A. L.: Some current trends in aphasia rehabilitation. Asha, 11:3-7, 1969.

Holland, A. L., and Matthews, J.: Application of teaching machine concepts to speech pathology and audiology. Asha, 5:474-482, 1963.

Honig, W. K. (Ed.): Operant Behavior: Areas of Research and Application. New York, Appleton-Century-Crofts, 1966.

Krasner, L., and Ullmann, L. P. (Eds.): Research in Behavior Modification. New York, Holt, Rinehart and Winston, 1965.

Lumsdaine, A. A., and Glaser, R. (Eds.): Teaching Machines and Programmed Learning. Washington, D. C., National Education Association of the United States, 1960.

McLean, J. E.: Private communication, 1969.

McLean, J. E.: Shifting Stimulus Control of Articulation Response by Operant Techniques. Unpublished doctoral dissertation, University of Kansas, 1965a.

McLean, J. E.: Extending stimulus control of phoneme articulation by operant techniques. In F. L. Girardeau and J. E. Spradlin (Eds.): ASHA Monographs Number 14, 1970.

McLean, J. E.: Shifting Stimulus Control of Articulation Responses by Operant Techniques, Parsons Demonstration Project, Report No. 82. Parsons, Parsons State Hospital, 1967.

McLean, J. E., and Spradlin, J.: Programming of Antecedent Stimulus Conditions in Operant Programs for Speech Modification, Parsons Demonstration Project, Report No. 87. Parsons, Parsons State Hospital, 1967.

Mager, R. F.: Preparing Objectives for Programmed Instruction. San Francisco, Fearon Publishers, 1962.

Rigg, K. E.: The Properant, Communications Research Laboratory Working Paper. Department of Speech, New Mexico State University, 1967.

Skinner, B. F.: The experimental analysis of behavior. Am Sci, 45:343-371, 1957a.

Skinner, B. F.: Reflections on a decade of teaching machines. In R. Glaser (Ed.): Teaching Machines and Programmed Learning, II. Washington, D. C., Department of Audiovisual Instruction, National Education Association of the United States, 1965.

Skinner, B. F.: Science and Human Behavior. New York, Macmillan, 1953.

Skinner, B. F.: The science of learning and the art of teaching. In A. A. Lumsdaine and R. Glaser (Eds.): Teaching Machines and Programmed Learning. Washington, D. C., National Education Association of the United States, 1960.

Skinner, B. F.: Teaching machines. Science, 128:969-977, 1958.

Skinner, B. F.: Verbal Behavior. New York, Appleton-Century-Crofts, 1957b.

Sloane, H. N., and MacAulay, B. D. (Eds.): Operant Procedures in Remedial Speech and Language Training. Boston, Houghton Mifflin, 1968.

Templin, M.: A study of sound discrimination ability in elementary school pupils. J Speech Hear Disord, 8:127-132, 1943.

Templin, M., and Darley, F. L.: The Templin-Darley Tests of Articulation. Iowa City, Bureau of Educational Research and Service, 1960.

Ulrich, R., Stachnik, T., and Mabry, J.: Control of Human Behavior. Glenview, Scott, Foresman, 1966.

Wolpe, J.: Psychotherapy by Reciprocal Inhibition. Palo Alto, Stanford University Press, 1958.

Wolpe, J., and Lazarus, A. A.: Behavior Therapy Techniques. New York, Pergamon Press, 1966.

Wolpe, J., Salter, A., and Reyna, L. J. (Eds.): The Conditioning Therapies. New York, Holt, Rinehart and Winston, 1964.

CHAPTER VII

A BEHAVIORISTIC APPROACH TO MODIFICATION OF ARTICULATION

DONALD E. MOWRER

DURING the past decade it has become increasingly apparent that learning principles derived from the behavioral sciences can be fruitfully applied to procedures employed in speech therapy. This chapter discusses a simplified behavior modification model and suggests its usefulness to the speech clinician.

The process of therapy undertaken within a behavioral model framework is predicated upon two sets of events: (1) *antecedent events*, which consist of instructions given by the speech clinician to evoke the desired behavior and (2) *consequent events*, which serve to strengthen or weaken the behavior which has been evoked. This process can be represented by a cycle which includes the antecedent event, the child's response and the consequent event. The cycle is repeated continuously until the instructional period is ended. Efficacy is determined by the number of cycles completed in a given time unit and the amount of actual behavioral change.

Completing this simple instructional model requires the addition of two basic principles: (1) identifying the behavior that is to be changed during the instructional process and (2) recording the extent of the behavioral change. By specifying the exact behavior which is to be altered and by keeping accurate records of behavioral change, the speech clinician greatly enhances the accountability of his therapy program.

In short, the basic procedure of behavioral modification consists

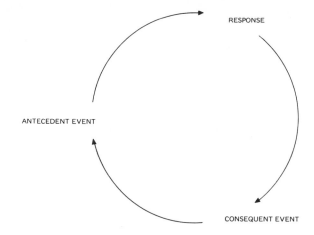

Figure VII-1. Instructional cycle.

of the following:
1. Select the target behavior to be changed.
2. Provide instructions to evoke the behavior.
3. Provide consequences to strengthen or weaken behaviors.
4. Keep records of response frequencies.

SELECT A TARGET BEHAVIOR FOR CHANGE

The first step in changing a behavior is to identify a specific behavioral target. To qualify as a behavioral target, two criteria must be met: (1) the behavior must be countable, and (2) it must be manipulatable, i.e. capable of being either increased or decreased.

Countable

The rule to follow in selecting a countable behavior is to state the behavior in such a way that someone else could count the behavior as you would. For example, to count the number of times the tongue protruded between the teeth during production of the /s/ would be an *observable* behavior which anyone could count. A distorted /ʒ/, while not observable to the eye, can be identified auditorily. Speech clinicians can learn to discriminate between occurrence of correct and incorrect / ʒ / productions. On the other hand, to speak with a *lazy tongue* would not be a behavior someone could count accurately, since there would be much disagreement concerning when the tongue was *lazy.*

Manipulatable

The observed behavior must be capable of being increased or decreased. Speech problems which consist of misarticulations usually include a behavior we wish to decrease, the error, and a behavior we want to increase, the correct sound. We also may wish to maintain or stabilize the frequency of a certain behavior. For example, we may wish to increase the frequency with which Billy uses / ʒ / correctly in words in connected speech. We may wish to decrease the frequency with which Mary allows air to escape laterally during /s/ production. Decreasing the frequency of nasal emission in the speech of a child who has a cleft hard palate may be impossible without surgical intervention or a prosthetic device so nasal emission may not be alterable using an instructional cycle alone.

Selecting a target behavior for change is usually accomplished by administering an articulation test. A wide variety of articulation proficiency tests are available. Some of these tests measure articulation skills in single words while others evaluate articulation proficiency via imitation, oral reading and conversational speech (Milisen *et al.,* 1954; Bradley, 1970). Using such multi-elicitation procedures, a speech clinician can identify specific behaviors to be modified. It is from such tests that the clinician formulates the first as well as the final behavioral objectives. For example, a first behavioral objective might be "to close the teeth while saying /s/ in isolation three times in rapid succession." A final objective might be "to use /s/ correctly in connected speech while talking to the teacher."

PROVIDE INSTRUCTIONS TO EVOKE THE BEHAVIOR: ANTECEDENT EVENTS

In order to obtain the desired speech behavior, the clinician must in some way provide a cue to the child, i.e. verbal, visual, kinesthetic, prosthetic, pictorial or textual. Cues can vary from very strong ones (which provide the child with a maximum amount of information with respect to how he should respond) to those containing minimal information. The cue, "Close your teeth like this and say /s/. Watch me do it a few times (demonstration). Now, I'll push on your chin to help you keep your teeth closed," contains verbal, visual and kinesthetic cues, whereas the cue, "Say /s/," is a weak verbal cue.

Mowrer (1971a) asked speech clinicians to identify cues which they found to be most successful for evoking /ʒ/. A total of 34 different cues were listed for the /ʒ/sound alone. A study by Chapman *et al.* (1961) revealed that 42 different procedures were suggested by speech clinicians as popular cuing instructions. It would appear that no single cue is adequate to evoke the desired response from all children. Speech clinicians appear to have favorite cues which they use first, and if unsuccessful, they resort to one of a variety of other cues from a hierarchial pattern.

In addition to the cue, the difficulty of the task to be performed must be considered as part of the antecedent event. Saying /s/ in isolation appears to be an easier task to perform than saying a word containing an /s/ blend in a sentence. Traditionally speech clinicians have taught the target sound in the following general task order: (1) isolation, (2) syllables, (3) words, (4) phrases, (5) sentences, (6) connected or conversational speech.

A programatic procedure for presenting instructional material can therefore be developed by carefully manipulating separate continua of cues and tasks. Tasks are arranged from easy to difficult; cues are listed from strong ones with maximum information to weak ones containing minimal supportive help.

The child who misarticulates a sound is presented with the easiest task (task 1), along with a strong cue (cue 1). Practice on task 1 is provided, and the cues are reduced in strength along the continuum from one to six until the child can produce the task behavior with minimal cues. When this criterion is reached, task 2 is presented. The strongest cue (cue 1) is presented at this time since there is maximum probability of failure when task difficulty is increased. Again, as the second task is practiced, the strength of

TABLE I

TASK AND CUE CONTINUUM

1	2	3	4	5	6

| easy | | moderate | | | difficult |

TASK

1	2	3	4	5	6

| strong | | moderate | | | weak |

CUE

the cue is again weakened until the child can perform the behavior with minimal cues. The final objective is reached when the child can perform task 6, which is speaking in various conditions without the aid of strong supportive cues.

There are two general program writing strategies which can be used as formats to present cues and tasks. One might be called a *stair-step* strategy. Each task is seen as an independent learning step. Consider, for example, task 1 as saying /s/ in isolation, task 2 saying /s/ in syllables and task 3 saying /s/ in the initial position of words. The first 20 instructional items develop and stabilize task 1; the next 15 items teach task 2. After the child learns task 1 to criterion, he is not asked to perform this task during any of the next 15 items in task 2. Likewise, when he masters task 2 he will not be asked to say /s/ in syllables again after he has moved to task 3. Thus, the task program moves in a stair-step, non-reviewing manner.

The second strategy is a *saw-tooth* task presentation. In this program, the child who is practicing task 2 will be asked to perform a few task-1 items for review. When he performs task 3 he also will practice some task-2 items, as well as a few task-1 items. The advantage of the saw-tooth program is that review items are built into it while the stair-step program moves successively from one task to the next.

In summary, two variables comprise the antecedent event of the instructional cycle: instructional cues and the level of task difficulty. They are interdependent. As a given task is practiced, cues decrease in strength; when task difficulty is increased, so is the strength of the cue.

PROVIDE CONSEQUENCES TO STRENGTHEN
OR WEAKEN BEHAVIOR

Much of the power inherent in the behavioral change model is found in the nature of the consequent event. The type of consequence occurring during or immediately after a behavior has a great deal to do with the future strength and direction of that behavior. The consequent event may serve to strengthen, to weaken or to have no effect upon the behavior. A strengthening consequence is one which increases the frequency of the behavior which immediately precedes it. Typical examples of strengthening consequences are statements of praise or various rewards in the form of toys, points, candy or money. A weakening consequence is one which decreases the frequency of the behavior which immediately precedes it. Statements such as "no," "you're wrong," "you missed it" are usually weakening consequents as are shock, loud buzzer sounds or other aversive sounds. Some consequences which we think would have an effect upon a behavior may have no effect whatever. This condition is fre-quently noted when working with children classified as autistic. With such children, social praise or candy often seem to have little effect upon behavior.

Using Consequences to Change Behavior

If the clinician wishes to increase the frequency of a behavior, he should use a strengthening consequence *immediately* following the desired behavior and use it *consistently.* The immediate use of a strengthening consequence has been shown to be a powerful determinant of future behaviors. As soon as the child says the sound correctly, the clinician should say, "Good," if social praise is the selected strengthening consequence. Waiting until the end of the session to tell a child he performed well may have no effect upon increasing the frequency of the desired behavior.

Using the consequence consistently has also been shown to be effective in increasing a behavior. The sporadic, random presentation of consequences is a poor way to build a weak behavior into a strong one. Only after the behavior is well established should a more random presentation of the consequences be used.

If the frequency of a response is to be decreased, use a weakening consequence immediately after the behavior and use it consistently. The weakening consequence may sometimes be a form of punishment. Again, the principles of immediacy and consistency are extremely important if the weakening consequence is to be effective.

A second way a behavior can be decreased is to evoke an incompatible behavior in place of the undesirable behavior. For example, if you instruct a lisping child to close his teeth when saying /s/, then the undesired tongue protrusion which normally occurs during /s/ production cannot occur. You strengthen the incompatible behavior and by doing so, weaken the undesirable behavior.

In short, if you wish to decrease the frequency of an unwanted speech behavior, you may (1) immediately and consistently present a weakening consequence following the undesirable behavior or (2) immediately and consistently present a strengthening consequence for some desired speech behavior which is incompatible with the unwanted behavior. A combination of both procedures can be used effectively to weaken behaviors.

Once a behavior has been increased, you may wish to maintain it at a certain level, to make it habitual. In other words, it is not the intent that the child say more /s/, / ʒ / or / θ / sounds. The intent is simply to increase the frequency of the correct sounds as opposed to the use of the incorrect sounds. In order to maintain the frequency of a behavior, use a strengthening consequence immediately but *inconsistently*. A consistent use of a strengthening consequence is critical to the establishment of a behavior, but the less frequent use of that consequence will serve to maintain the behavior once it has been well established. Some of our most persistent behaviors receive strengthening consequences only periodically. An example of this kind of maintenance is found among those who sell items door-to-door. A sale to every sixth to tenth housewife is usually sufficient to keep a salesman ringing doorbells all day.

After a child demonstrates adequate mastery of a task, the strengthening consequence can be given following every other correct response, then following every third or fourth correct response. When a more difficult task is presented, the strengthening consequence can be given continuously again and faded out as the task is mastered. During the final stages of therapy the strengthening consequence is rarely used and finally, it is terminated altogether. It should be observed, however, that if reduction of the strengthening consequence occurs too rapidly, the desired response may weaken considerably. A summary of the effects of consequent events is presented in Table II.

Strengthening Consequences

There are many consequent events which serve to increase behavior frequency. It should be stressed that the child's behavior tells us whether or not a consequence is strengthening. If the frequency of the correct response decreases the consequence is a weakener, regardless of what we think it should be. Often classroom teachers punish children for leaving their seats by scolding them immediately upon seat-leaving. By keeping records, it may be found that seat-leaving behavior in some children actually increases under these consequences. The teacher's scolding is a weakener by *her definition*, but it is by *observation* a strengthener. The teacher's scolding is a form of attention which

TABLE II

EFFECTS OF CONSEQUENT EVENTS

BEHAVIOR DIRECTION	KIND OF CONSEQUENCE	WHEN TO ADMINISTER	HOW OFTEN TO ADMINISTER
Increase	Strengthening	Immediately	Consistently
Decrease	Weakening	Immediately	Consistently
Decrease	Strengthening an incompatible behavior	Immediately	Consistently
Maintain	Strengthening	Immediately	Inconsistently

acts as a strengthening consequence to some children, but since scolding acts as a weakening consequence to most children the teacher continues to use it, even though scolding actually increases the behavior the teacher wishes to decrease.

There are several ways that strengthening consequences can be identified. One is to observe the child to discover what are his preferred activities. If a child frequently visits the desk of his teacher, then teacher recognition may be the strengthening consequence. For some, reading comic books is a preferred activity; others prefer to draw pictures and seek drawing materials. On the other hand, if the child is observed to be solving math problems, this behavior might be the result of the teacher's preference, not the child's. As soon as the teacher leaves the scene, he stops doing math problems. Aside from observing the child's preferred activities, the clinician may ask the child what he would like. Questions like, "What school supplies would you like to have?" or "What would you like to be able to do in school that you usually don't get to do?" often reveal strengthening consequences. Teachers are often very perceptive regarding things children like to get or like to do and can quickly list many strengthening consequences. Parents also can help identify what could be used as strengthening consequences for their children.

When a variety of consequences have been identified, they can be compiled into a list from which a child can choose.* Once he has chosen an item or a favorite activity, an agreement is created between the clinician and the child. The clinician sets a goal for the child to accomplish and defines what the child must do to achieve the goal (i.e. say /s/ correctly in 24 words containing /s/ in the final position). In return the child agrees to work toward achieving the goal for some item on the reinforcement list.

A convenient procedure for measuring out a strengthening consequence "a little at a time" is to use a *token system.* This system might consist simply of making a slash mark on paper each time the child says the sound correctly. After the child has earned a specified number of points, he is entitled to the strengthening consequence of his choice. A single cartoon cut from a Peanuts pocket cartoon book might cost 100 points. A piece of red construction paper might cost 200 points, whereas 500 points might be required for a new wooden pencil.

Some children may wish to save their points in much the same manner as many housewives save trading stamps. It is often wise to select a coupon or token ratio plan so the child can save large amounts of points easily. Often a child will save 300-500 points during a single twenty-minute therapy session. If one coupon is given per 100 points, then the point redemption process becomes much easier to manage and easier for the child to comprehend. The child may carry a *coupon card* containing 50 triangles. The clinician places a 0 in a triangle when 100 correct sounds have been said. The strengthening consequences found on the list are each assigned a certain number of *triangle* values. When the child presents his triangle card for an item on the list, the clinician checks them off (the appropriate number of triangles) by placing an X in the 0 which was placed in the earned triangle.

The above scoring system can be altered in a number of ways, dependent only upon the imagination and resourcefulness of the clinician. In conducting research for my doctoral dissertation, I used small plastic chips about the size of a penny. These chips

*Reinforcement items which have been used by clinicians include: colored construction paper, pencils, seeds to plant, cartoons cut from comic books, having a friend for supper, having the clinician carry his lunch tray, etc.

were dispensed into a clear plastic container (Mowrer, 1964). When a number of chips had been dispensed up to a red line marked on the container, the child was entitled to receive a small plastic toy. By keeping the chips out of the child's reach, the distractive features of manipulating the chips were reduced.

Regardless of the method employed, an effective token economy system should include the following:

1. The token should be dispensed with minimum effort immediately following a correct response.
2. The tokens should not interfere with learning the task.
3. The child should be able to exchange the tokens for something which he desires.
4. There should be much earning and spending of tokens, i.e. an active economy.

Weakening Consequences

The most widespread weakening consequence is a verbal statement to the effect that the child was wrong. Such statements as "No," "That's not right," "You missed it," accompanied by slight frowns, head shaking and general disapproval are weakening consequences which are used frequently. A buzzer sounded immediately following an incorrect response may also serve as a weakener if this consequence is explained to the child beforehand. Electric shock has also been used as a weakener in some laboratory studies involving people who stutter. Silence or just ignoring an incorrect response often acts as a weakening consequence. If a token system is being used, a token is not delivered following an incorrect response. Grey (1970) recommends this procedure for dealing with incorrect responses children make while being instructed in his program of language acquisition through programmed conditioning. If two or more children are being taught simultaneously, unwanted behaviors of one child can be reduced by presenting tokens to another member in the group who is not producing the undesirable behavior. For example, if three children are in group therapy and Child A continues talking out of turn, give extra tokens to those who do not talk out of turn.

Another effective means of controlling undesirable behavior is to withdraw a token immediately following an undesirable behavior. Great care should be used with this type of consequence since many children strongly resent losing something they have earned. Conley (1966) demonstrated the effectiveness of token withdrawal by telling a small group of peers that when the experimental subject said /s/ correctly each would receive a token. However, when the subject said /s/ incorrectly, each member would lose a token. Experimental subjects in the group Conley studied made significantly fewer errors than did a similar group who did not lose tokens contingent upon errors. Withdrawing tokens should probably be reserved for errors produced after the instructional program is well underway rather than during the acquisition phase of task learning.

Finally, a last-resort procedure found most effective in controlling very disruptive behaviors is called *time-out*. The child is removed from the instructional setting for one or more minutes contingent upon undesirable behavior. The speech clinician will probably not choose this weakening consequence for speech errors but may wish to use it occasionally as a means of controlling disruptive behaviors. Time-out simply removes the child from the situation in which he could earn tokens. The area outside the speech therapy room may serve as the time-out quarters.

In summary, incorrect articulation responses can be decreased by (1) telling the child he is wrong, (2) ignoring incorrect responses, (3) presenting an aversive stimulus (a buzzer or withdrawal of token) immediately following the incorrect response or (4) strengthening an incompatible behavior. Detrimental disruptive behavior often can be brought under control using a time-out contingency.

KEEPING RECORDS OF BEHAVIOR CHANGE

By keeping accurate records, the speech clinician can learn much about both his instructional program and the effects of the consequent events he has chosen. The data gathered from daily records also become valuable when he is asked to account for his time. School principals are interested in the speech improvement of children over a given time period, as well as in the costs involved in correcting speech problems. Only by keeping accurate records can these facts be known.

If a token economy system is used, three-fourths of the record keeping work is already finished. The clinician need only determine response rate per minute and record these data on a graph. Calculation of response rate requires that the therapy session be timed. If the child has earned 240 points during a 20 minute therapy session, correct response rate per minute can be determined by dividing 20 into 240 yielding a quotient of 12 responses per minute. This number can be plotted on a graph. The error rate is computed by dividing 20 into the total number of errors, say in this case 80 yielding a quotient of 4. This number is also plotted on the graph. The total response rate is determined in a like manner (therapy time divided into total number of responses).

Two methods of graphing have been used to record these data: a linear graph and a logarithmic graph form. The linear graph portrays increases in frequency as equal intervals vertically. The logarithmic graph displays frequency increases in equal proportions. For example, on a logarithmic graph increasing the frequency of a behavior from 2 to 4 (a 100% increase) is shown as the same amount of increase as an increase of from 30 to 60 (also a 100% increase). These same increases would be displayed quite differently on a linear graph. The distance from 2 to 4 would be small whereas an increase from 30 to 60 would be represented by a large distance between points. The merits of using a logarithmic graph in favor of the linear graph to represent speech responses have been discussed elsewhere (Mowrer, 1969b, 1971b).

By observing changes in the frequency total responses and error responses, the clinician can analyze therapy sessions objectively. If total response frequency decreases radically, the clinician should question the value of the instructional activity to determine if the activity depressed response frequency. If frequency of the error response increases, the clinician may wish to revert to an easier task or increase the strength of the cues being used. Changing the consequent event schedule may also help to reduce errors. If a token system is being used on an intermittent basis, the schedule could be changed to a continuous one, or two tokens could be given following each correct response instead of just one token. By graphing response frequency data, the clinician is provided with important information that can help him make his instructional program more effective.

Bradley (1970) prefers to keep records of instructional sessions on a table rather than on a graph. Session dates are recorded in the left hand column. The sound being taught is recorded under one of five task headings depending upon which task is being taught. Response frequencies are recorded in the columns on the right hand side of the table. When the child reaches the criterion stated by the clinician, the child is advanced to the next task. In Table III, data from a therapy session conducted at Arizona State University are presented concerning one child who was being taught /k/ and /f/ sounds. Such a table allows the clinician to know at a glance which tasks the child has mastered, how many minutes were required to master the tasks and which task should be practiced during the next therapy session. By knowing the cost of therapy time on a per hour basis, it is possible to assign direct costs to the correction of each sound as well as the cost of mastering each task.

Some general guidelines have been established with regard to response frequencies one should expect during speech therapy. Hurley (1969) indicated that public school clinicians that she studied evoked from a low of .58 target responses per minute to a high of 6.0 responses per minute. The mean rate was 2.79 responses for the 10 therapy sessions studied. An analysis of S–PACK revealed a mean response rate of over 7 target /s/ responses per minute during the three session clinic program (Mowrer, Baker and Schutz, 1970). Clinicians should expect response frequency to be high during the initial stages of therapy when the target phoneme is being evoked in isolation or in words and to decrease as phrase and sentence contexts are introduced. Initial response frequencies should average between 15 to 25 per minute and taper down to 6 to 10 responses during connected speech.

A general guideline for the frequency of error rate was provided in a study of the correction of the frontal lisp (Mowrer, 1964). It was found that children whose error rate while being instructed in

TABLE III

TABLE FOR RECORDING RESPONSE FREQUENCY

PATIENT ___Chuck___   Date _____

CLINICIAN ___Calhoun___

ARTICULATION DATA SHEET

Date	Session	Activity							Time	Tot. Resp.	Tot. Error	Tot. Corr.	% Corr.	Comments
			Iso.	Syl.	Words	Sent.	Read.	Conv.						
2-19	1		K						10	55	15	40	73	Last 10 R=100%
2-22	2			K					40	417	69	348	84	
2-24	3			K					15	150	6	144	96	
					K				10	145	22	123	85	in initial position
2-26	4		F						6.	80	6	74	93	
			F						8	90	2	88	97	
3-1	5				K				24	380	28	352	93	in initial position
						K			15	230	20	210	91	phrases "the cook"
				F					15	200	2	198	99	
									143	1737	170	1567	90%	

therapy sessions was below 20 per cent produced /s/ correctly on 90 per cent of the 30 criterion test items while children whose error rate was above 20 per cent scored less than 50 per cent on the criterion test. From these data one might conclude that the child whose error rate is greater than 20 per cent during the instructional period may not be profiting from the instructional program. If the child's error rate climbs over 20 per cent this might serve as an indication for the clinician to take immediate steps toward reducing error rate by increasing cues and/or decreasing task difficulty.

Unless records of correct and incorrect responses are kept, one has only a vague notion of the frequency of errors. Analysis of the error rate of one therapy session conducted by a student clinician revealed the error rate of a five-year-old child was 87 per cent (Mowrer, 1969a). The clinician knew that the session was not progressing smoothly, but he had no idea the child was experiencing failure to this degree. Further analysis of the therapy session revealed that the child's disruptive behaviors (dropping his pencil, asking to leave the session, playing with the tokens, etc.) increased 60 per cent during the second half of the session. High error rates may in some cases lead to the development of discipline problems.

In summary, keeping records of responses and graphing response frequencies help the clinician to determine the effects of the consequences being used (consequent events) and to make relevant changes in the instructional program (antecedent events). Keeping records also permits the clinician to make accurate cost estimates of therapy services since time can be related to behavior change.

The four basic components of the behavioral model comprise the essentials of *precision teaching* in speech therapy. The use of the behavioral model framework provides the speech clinician with an effective system into which an instructional program can be implanted. Precision comes as the clinician receives feedback from response data and takes steps to improve upon the instructional program.

REFERENCES

Bradley, Doris: Articulation programs. Technical report presented at the workshop on operant analysis of communication problems, Taos, New Mexico, 1970.

Chapman, M., Hebert, E., Avery, C., and Selmar, J.: Clinical practice: remedial procedures. J Speech Hear Disord, Monograph Supplement 8:58-77, 1961.

EPRA, Reinforcement display panel LC-2. Tempe, Arizona, 1968.

Grey, Burl: Language problems: language acquisition through programmed conditioning. In Robert Bradfield, (Ed.): Behavior Modification: The Human Effort. San Rafael, Dimensions Publishing, 1970.

Hurley, M.: Measuring clinician competency. In D. E. Mowrer, (Ed.): Modification of Speech Behaviors: Ideas and Strategies for Students. Tempe, Arizona State University Bookstore, 1969.

Milisen, R. *et al.:* The disorder of articulation: a systematic clinical and experimental approach. J Speech Hear Disord, Monograph Supplement 4:1-86, 1954.

Mowrer, D. E.: An experimental analysis of variables controlling lisping responses of children. Ph.D. dissertation, Arizona State University, 1964.

Mowrer, D. E. (Ed.): Modification of Speech Behavior: Ideas and Strategies for Students. Tempe, Arizona State University Bookstore, 1969a.

Mowrer, D. E.: Evaluating speech therapy through precision recording. J Speech Hear Disord, 34:239-244, 1969b.

Mowrer, D. E.: Technical report # 6: evoking /ʒ/. SWRL differentiated speech project. Inglewood, 1971a.

Mowrer, D. E., Baker, R., and Schutz, R.: S–PACK: Modification of the Frontal Lisp, EPRA, Tempe, 1970.

Mowrer, D. E.: Developing Precision in Recording Speech Behaviors. Salt Lake City, Word Making Productions, 1971b.

CHAPTER VIII

A THEORETICAL AND OPERATIONAL ANALYSIS OF THE PAIRED STIMULI TECHNIQUE

JOHN V. IRWIN and FRANCIS A. GRIFFITH

T HE *Paired-Stimuli Technique* for the modification of articulatory errors, described by Weston and Irwin (1971), is an attempt to provide rapid, efficient treatment of articulatory deviations, with a particular view toward reducing intervention time in the school setting. The procedures are based on the assumption that specific phonemic responses within a subject's repertoire (or which can be established with minimal teaching) can be generalized to other phonetic contexts. That is, an effort is made to locate a word in which the subject produces his target phoneme acceptably; such a word is designated as a key word. In the technique, the subject produces this word alternately with ten other words in which the target phoneme is produced unacceptably; such words are called training words. Tangible reinforcers are given on a continuous (100%) schedule for socially acceptable production of the target phoneme, whether it occurs in the key

NOTE: The work reported in this chapter was supported in part by the United States Office of Education, Bureau of Education for the Handicapped and by the Department of Audiology and Speech Pathology, Memphis State University, through funds made available under Title VI.

The authors express their sincere appreciation to Drs. Alan J. Weston and Donald L. Rampp, who were instrumental in the planning and administration of the pilot study as conducted in Mississippi and Arkansas, respectively. Our thanks are also offered to Mrs. Cheri Resler and Miss Ann Daniel, who supervised the collection of data reported from the pilot study.

word or a training word. This pairing procedure continues until criterion is reached. Criterion is defined as socially acceptable production of the target phoneme under conditions of no reinforcement in at least eight of the ten training words over two successive sessions. The target phoneme is trained to criterion in only one position (initial or final) of a word at a time. If the target phoneme is misarticulated in both initial and final positions of words, criterion must be met twice, once for each position. Each of these definitions and procedures is elaborated later in this chapter.

CRITERIA FOR AN EFFECTIVE ARTICULATORY INTERVENTION PROGRAM IN THE SCHOOLS

It may be helpful to frame potential criteria for an effective articulatory intervention program in the schools for at least two reasons. First, they can guide the creative clinician in the modification of those techniques that are now available to him. Second, they can serve as guidelines against which present intervention techniques can be evaluated. These criteria for an effective program of articulatory modification arose from an interest in the modification of phonological deviations, both articulatory and phonatory. The extension of the criteria to other types of deviations may not be in order. With this in mind, it is convenient — and probably realistic — to subsume the criteria for an effective articulatory intervention program under three headings: subjects, method and results. The *Paired-Stimuli Technique* represents a deliberate effort to satisfy the criteria discussed under each of these headings.

Subjects

Polyphonemic. An effective method should be applicable to any phonological deviation. With reference to articulatory behavior, to which the *Paired-Stimuli Technique* is addressed, it should be polyphonemic. That is, it should be applicable to subjects who misarticulate few sounds and to those who misarticulate many. In practice, this method has been demonstrated to be effective with subjects who misarticulate various consonant sounds. The applicability of the technique to subjects whose primary misarticulation pattern consists of vowel errors has not been demonstrated.

Wide Range and Ability. An effective method should be usable with an age range from young children through adults. Attention should be paid to the stimulus materials appropriate to the skills associated with certain ages, e.g. it should be usable with subjects who cannot read. The *Paired-Stimuli Technique* satisfies this criterion by virtue of its current use of picture stimuli, but more broadly by its adaptability to use with other stimulus materials.

Independent of Etiology. It is extremely difficult to diagnose articulation problems in the medical-model sense of isolating a cause which is the proper focus of treatment. Even if such diagnosis were possible, the presumed consequences of certain disorders may not justify its cost in terms of time and personnel. For these reasons, a method that offers a high probability of success, irrespective of etiological factors, is desirable. Like most behavior modification programs, the *Paired-Stimuli Technique* relies upon behavioral baselines for its use, without regard for the etiology of the behaviors.

Self-Screening. Finally, since children would be put into such a program on the basis of observed articulatory deviations without diagnosis, it is imperative that the method be self-screening. Self-screening, as the term is used here, implies screening at two points in time. First, it should be possible to establish simple behavioral criteria that will serve as a guide for inclusion or exclusion of subjects relative to the program. Second, after inclusion of a subject, the method should provide quick, objective evidence of his success or failure. The *Paired-Stimuli Technique* satisfies both of these criteria. The first criterion is met by the administration of any articulatory test battery (Irwin, 1971b) and by determination that a subject (1) has some spontaneous speech and (2) is able to produce his target phoneme acceptably in at least one word, either prior to, or as the result of, therapy. Evidence of success or failure after a subject's inclusion in the program is defined in terms of established criteria for the termination of intervention and by appropriate measures of generalization.

Method

No Specialized Equipment. Inasmuch as the intent in the development of the *Paired-Stimuli Technique* was to provide a method that would be useful in mass modification programs in the schools, the use of specialized equipment should be avoided. Cost, portability, maintenance and space are all factors which frequently mitigate against the use of specialized equipment. The *Paired-Stimuli Technique* can be used with materials improvised by the clinician for particular clients, but for clinical convenience a *Paired-Stimuli Kit* has been developed for commercial distribution.

Consistency of Program Format. In order for clinicians to use a technique with a wide range of articulatory deviations, it seems essential that the same basic program be applicable to each deviation. Furthermore, it would be desirable for the basic intervention plan to continue unchanged when criterion is reached on a particular phoneme. In short, the simpler and more repetitive the program format, the easier it would be to teach clinicians to use it precisely and for clients to understand and respond to it appropriately. The *Paired-Stimuli Technique* employs one basic program for all articulatory defects through all stages of improvement.

Potentially Usable by Sub-Professionals. In order to reduce costs and increase services, it would be desirable for an effective articulatory intervention program to be usable by sub-professionals (clinical aides). A total intervention program requires the administration and interpretation of appropriate tests of articulation and the planning of a sequence of sounds to be modified, in addition to the administration of the intervention program itself. If all of these duties are to be assumed by one person, the skills of a trained speech pathologist are ordinarily required. However, once the identification of subjects and the planning of their programs has been completed by a speech clinician, it is feasible for a trained clinical aide to carry out the *Paired-Stimuli* intervention program, under the supervision of the speech clinician. The primary qualifications for effective use of the intervention program are (1) comprehension of all procedures, (2) good ability to discriminate socially acceptable productions of the target phoneme and (3) the ability to make reliable judgments of acceptability, so that appropriate positive reinforcement is provided for the subject.

Intrinsic Motivation. Holding young children's interest in therapeutic activities is sometimes a problem. Many speech clinicians stimulate children's interest by using activities which may divert the activity's intended purpose. For example, many clinicians use games which arouse children's competitiveness, but the end-goal of the children's achieving better speech production may be diminished by their immediate interest in winning or in the mechanics of the game. The *Paired-Stimuli Technique* employs 100 per cent contingent positive reinforcement for socially acceptable production of the target phoneme in a key word and/or a training word. Reinforcement is in the form of tokens, which are redeemable for back-up reinforcers such as candy, toys or money. Token reinforcers tend to maintain children's interest in the therapeutic activity because each child competes only with himself and because his "pay-off" (back-up reinforcers) is never related to chance. The number of tokens a child earns each day is the direct result of his acceptable performance of the target behavior.

Results

Rapid Achievement of Goals. An effective method of articulatory intervention for use in the schools should permit rapid acquisition of the desired target behavior. Satisfaction of this criterion would mean that: (1) Each child would be kept out of the classroom for a relatively short period of time for the remediation of his difficulties. Obviously, this would be desirable from the academic standpoint, especially since many children with speech and/or language problems may also have academic difficulties. (2) More children could be treated and dismissed from therapy as having made maximal improvement. Thus, a greater number of children could be treated during each school year. Because of our profession's recent involvement with language deviations and learning disabilities, rapid termination of articulation cases might make it possible to spend more time working with these and other groups of children. (3) Children could be seen for articulatory therapy who, by virtue of their age and specific phonemic deviations, might ordinarily not be treated on the assumption that their errors would be self-correcting over time. Possible erroneous prediction of self-correction – and the potential negative consequences for the child of such erroneous prediction – could be minimized or eliminated because these questionable children could be treated effectively and rapidly.

Evidence reported later in this chapter indicates that the *Paired-Stimuli Technique* is very rapid in achievement of its goals and that its application on a large scale in school settings would make advantages such as those noted above possible of realization.

Good Generalization. No method of articulatory intervention can be considered successful unless it (1) leads directly to good generalization in real-life speaking situations or (2) provides a systematic base for the use of other techniques which, in turn, accomplish such generalization. Evidence presented in Table XI, *Screening Deep Test* (McDonald) by *Data Collection Interval* and *Phoneme Category,* supports the conclusion that the *Paired-Stimuli Technique* leads to good generalization in the type of word contexts sampled in this test. Evidence is less conclusive – but very hopeful – that generalization to spontaneous speech also results from the *Paired-Stimuli* procedures. At present, refinements in the technique which may increase its potential for generalization to conversational speech are being explored. Also – and perhaps more importantly – methods for reliable prediction of generalization to conversational speech are being investigated.

No Negative Side Effects. For reasons already indicated, the assumption has been made that an effective intervention program should deal with behavior rather than with presumed causes. The *Paired-Stimuli Technique,* as is true of any such program, is subject to the possibility of producing effects other than those desired. The issue of symptom substitution as it relates to behavior modification has been reviewed by Irwin (1971a). With respect to the conversion symptom, Irwin stated

> The theory, then, is quite clear. Certain types of maladaptive behavior, that may easily include both receptive and expressive disorders of communication, may be symptoms of underlying conflicts. In such instances, resolution of the symptom is not

sufficient. The underlying or basic cause must be eliminated. (p. 19).

But the symptom conversion theory has not had acceptance by behavior therapists. Eysenck (1960) stated

> Learning theory does not postulate any such 'unconscious causes,' but regards neurotic symptoms as simply learned habits; there is no neurosis underlying the symptom, but merely the symptom itself. *Get rid of the symptom and you have eliminated the neurosis.* (p. 9).

The literature of communicative disorders recognizes the conversion symptom and its possible effects. In audiology, such standard texts as those by Newby (1964), O'Neill and Oyer (1966), Sataloff (1966) and Davis and Silverman (1970) explicitly recognize the existence of this mechanism. In speech pathology, writers such as Moses (1954), Perkins (1957), Van Riper (1957), Rousey and Moriarty (1965), Aronson (1969) and Murphy (1970) have dealt with the issue of the conversion symptom.

Evidence now seems fairly conclusive that the *Paired-Stimuli Technique* has minimal effects on speech sounds other than the target phoneme, as indicated by the failure of untreated phonemes to change as a function of training on a specific phoneme. Data pertinent to this issue are presented in Table XI.

The *Paired-Stimuli Technique* modifies behavior directly; it does not treat causes. To the extent that a clinician regards a subject's articulatory deviation as a symptom of underlying psychic conflict, then the use of this technique is potentially dangerous. The present authors, therefore, raise the topic of symptom substitution as an area of legitimate concern. On the basis of observation and parental reports to date, we have no evidence of this effect.

RATIONALE FOR LEARNING PRINCIPLES EMPLOYED IN THE PAIRED-STIMULI TECHNIQUE

Reward and Punishment

Theoretically, as has been noted in the early writings of Thorndike (1911) concerning the Law of Effect, reward (positive reinforcement) and punishment may be viewed as equal but opposite modifiers of behavior. According to Azrin and Holz (1966)

> The present definition of a punishing stimulus is identical to the definition of a reinforcing stimulus in that it requires a change in the future probability of a response resulting from the production of the stimulus by the response. The definitions differ only with respect to the direction of change of the response probability: an increase of probability for positive reinforcement, a decrease for punishment. Neither process is secondary to the other. (p. 383).

Table I, *A Theoretical Conception of Reward and Punishment*, presents this concept in a somewhat simplified form. As shown in the table, positive reinforcement, or reward, is defined as a stimulus which decreases the rate of a specified behavior. Both reward and punishment can modify behavior by their contingent addition or removal. In reward, as indicated in the table by blocks 1 and 3, behavior may be accelerated by adding a positive reinforcer, such as food, contingently or removing a stimulus, such

TABLE I

A THEORETICAL CONCEPTION OF REWARD
AND PUNISHMENT

REWARD	PUNISHMENT
1 Add Food, Money, Etc.	2 Add Electroshock, Noise, Etc.
3 Remove Electroshock, Noise, Etc.	4 Remove Food, Money, Etc.
ACCELERATE	DECELERATE

as electroshock, contingently. Again, as shown in blocks 2 and 4, punishment is exemplified by the contingent addition of a stimulus such as electroshock, or the contingent removal of a positive reinforcer, such as food.

As already stated, reward and punishment may be seen as theoretically equivalent in their power to modify behavior. However, a reveiw of the literature tends to minimize the value of punishment. Both Thorndike (1931) and Skinner (1948, 1953) have strongly denied the efficacy of punishment as compared with reward. On the basis of their statements, blocks 2 and 4 of Table I would be declared *off limits* to the clinician. Solomon (1963), in his presidential address to *The Eastern Psychological Association,* was less negative than Thorndike (1931) and Skinner (1948, 1953) with respect to punishment. Solomon took the position that no general claim could reasonably be made about its usefulness and that the efficacy of punishment must be evaluated in terms of a specific application in a specific learning situation. Even Solomon (1963), however, treated the technique with the following caution

> ... to conclude ... that the punishment procedure is typically either effective or ineffective, typically either a temporary suppressor or a permanent one, is to oversimplify irresponsibly a complex area of scientific knowledge, one still containing a myriad of intriguing problems for experimental attack. (p. 243).

As summarized in Table II, *An Interpretation of Response Rate Decelerators,* Azrin and Holz (1966) have compared punishment with other techniques. The techniques originally listed include *Extinction, Stimulus Variation, Restraint, Satiation* and *Punishment.* The present authors have added *Negative Practice.* The factors of comparison concern each technique's immediacy, its enduring effect, its completeness and its irreversibility. The reader will note that in Azrin and Holz's table (1966) as modified by the present authors, only punishment meets each of the criteria for an ideal response decelerator. Recognizing that Azrin and Holz's review is an interpretation of the literature, why is the status of punishment so low in the scientific community? At least two factors seem to account for it. First, it is difficult to predict the precise manner in which punishment will function in any given situation. As noted by Azrin and Holz (1966)

TABLE II

AN INTERPRETATION OF RESPONSE RATE DECELERATORS

TECHNIQUE	*IMMEDIATE EFFECT*	*ENDURING EFFECT*	*COMPLETE SUPPRESSION*	*IRREVERSIBLE EFFECT*
Extinction	No	Yes	No	No
Stimulus Variation	Yes	No	No	No
Restraint	Yes	Yes	Yes	No
Satiation	Yes	Yes	No	No
Negative Practice*	No	No?	No	No
Punishment	Yes	Yes	Yes	Yes

(After Azrin & Holz, 1966)

*Added by the present authors.

Perhaps the most paradoxical and confusing aspect of punishment has been the ability of a punishing stimulus to become a discriminative or conditioned reinforcing stimulus. This confusion arises when we fail to remember that a punishing stimulus is still a stimulus; as such, it can be inadvertently associated with reinforcing stimuli, with periods of reinforcement, with periods of extinction, and with other punishing stimuli. The result of such selective temporal association may be to strengthen, to neutralize, or even to reverse the aversive aspect of the punishing stimulus. (p. 442).

A second major objection relates to the possible negative side effects of punishment. The reader will note that negative side effects is not a heading in the modified Azrin and Holz (1966) table. But various investigators (Weiner, 1964; Azrin and Holz, 1966; Sajwaj, 1969; McReynolds and Huston, 1971; Griffith,

1971) have addressed themselves to this topic. It should be noted that negative side effects, as used here, may relate to effects on the clinician as well as on the subject.

A further objection to the use of punishment can be raised from the practical standpoint. Typically, most teacher-clinicians do not wish to punish their pupils. Our society imposes social penalties upon persons, other than parents, who punish children. With this in mind, it is likely that an intervention program based upon punishment procedures would be regarded as objectionable by many clinicians. Even if it were not repugnant to individual clinicians, the possibility of obtaining parental consent for the use of punishment with school children seems rather bleak. Finally, it is difficult to use punishment in situations where a client comes voluntarily for treatment because he always has the option of terminating because of the aversive nature of the program.

Recent experimentation within the field of speech pathology has suggested that contingent removal of a positive reinforcer, as indicated in block 4 of Table I, may be an effective and socially acceptable technique of punishment which may contribute to the acquisition of desired behaviors. The terms, token loss or response cost, have been used to describe the contingent removal of tokens used as positive reinforcers in order to eliminate undesired behaviors. McReynolds and Huston (1971) and Griffith (1971) have employed this technique with some success. But in both of these studies it was found that positive reinforcement was superior to alternating punishment conditions for the acquisition of imitative speech behaviors. Token loss studies directed toward the acquisition of articulatory behaviors also have a built-in problem when conceived for use on a large scale. As Azrin and Holz (1966) have observed " . . . some level of positive reinforcement must be made available in order to provide the opportunity for experimentally withdrawing that reinforcement." (p. 392). Finally, Azrin and Holz (1966) have answered the question of whether faster learning is produced by punishment or by reward as follows:

> The question has often been raised whether punishment is more or less effective than reward in teaching new behavior. This question has no meaning if we abide by the technical definition of punishment since punishment is a method of eliminating behavior whereas

reinforcement is a method of producing or maintaining behavior. (p. 430).

For the reasons noted above, punishment was rejected as a desirable and practical method for use in the training of socially acceptable articulatory behavior. Reward, and specifically the type presented in block 1 of Table I, was the method of choice. In this situation, something that is presumably desired is provided as a consequence of the subject's emitting the target behavior, with the intent of accelerating that behavior. Because of their ability to act as generalized reinforcers (Birnbrauer, Wolf, Kidder and Teague, 1965), tokens are used as positive reinforcers because they can be redeemed for a variety of objects or privileges. Thus, as presently employed, blocks 2, 3, and 4, as shown in Table I, are not utilized as a regular part of the *Paired-Stimuli Technique.* However, further research may indicate that certain of these alternatives are useful in conjunction with the *Paired-Stimuli* training procedures.

Acceleration Techniques

In Table III, *Major Techniques for Accelerating Behaviors,* Trial-and-Error and Insight are drawn from classical experimental

TABLE III

MAJOR TECHNIQUES FOR ACCELERATING BEHAVIORS

Trial-and-Error
Insight

Instruction
Stimulus Variation
Shaping
Building
Fading
Imitation

Expansion
Modeling
Prompting
Echoing

psychology. Thorndike (1913) espoused trial-and-error; Kohler (1925), insight. Spence (1951) has reviewed selected implications of this distinction. Current theorists tend to minimize the difference in the two techniques. Harlow (1967), for example, in his address to the luncheon of the forty-third annual convention of the *American Speech and Hearing Association,* suggested that the two are really not separate and that insight occurs primarily after previous trial and error.

Instruction, Stimulus Variation, Shaping, Building, Fading and *Imitation* are drawn from classical learning theory. In situations oriented toward operant concepts, the techniques of shaping and building have been particularly powerful and will be discussed later. *Expansion, Modeling, Prompting* and *Echoing* have been used in contemporary linguistic research. Of these, modeling and expansion have probably been the most significant.

Shaping is an operant technique that has been discussed by Sloane and MacAulay (1968) with specific reference to its use in speech pathology. In shaping, approximations of the desired terminal behavior are differentially reinforced, with the result that successive behaviors are gradually modified until they achieve the precise format desired. Shaping is a powerful technique, but its application in articulatory therapy is not easy because of the need to designate intermediate steps between the baseline and the terminal behaviors which can be judged reliably and quickly.

In *building,* only the specified response is reinforced; approximations are not. The advantage of building, obviously, is its rapidity. According to Brookshire (1967),

> Perhaps the simplest problems which face the speech clinician are those in which the responses of concern are present in the repertoire of the client before treatment is begun, and where the goal of the clinician is to increase or decrease the frequency of those responses in certain stimulus situations. (p. 222)

In explaining the procedures of building, Brookshire (1967) reported

> Clinical procedures in problems involving changes in rate of responding basically include structuring the situation so that the response of interest is emitted, and presenting a reinforcer to the client immediately following the response . . . (p. 222).

The possible disadvantage to building, as opposed to shaping, is the fact that the response must be in the subject's repertoire, even if at a very low rate.

With regard to the *Paired-Stimuli Technique,* the use of building assumes not only that the desired response is present intermittently, but also that the target·phoneme in the various training words is the same as the target phoneme in the key word. In any rigorous sense, this assumption of sameness is inaccurate. But the concept that the various target behaviors fall in the same response class is less difficult to accept. Indeed, the concept of the phoneme may serve to resolve this difficulty.

The literature on articulatory acquisition, as cited by Irwin (1971d), refers frequently to the instability both of error and correct articulatory production. Table IV, *Articulatory Responses by Children Categorized as Having a Specific Error Phoneme,* is drawn from three studies reported by Minifie, Burkhart and Wentland (1966). Each of these studies illustrated inconsistency in error phoneme production. Deep testing techniques such as those developed by McDonald (1964, 1968) represent methods of locating phonetic environments in which the desired response —

TABLE IV

ARTICULATORY RESPONSES BY CHILDREN CATEGORIZED
AS HAVING A SPECIFIC ERROR PHONEME

ERROR PHONEME	*NUMBER OF SUBJECTS*	*NUMBER OF TRIALS*	*NUMBER RIGHT*	*PER CENT RIGHT*
r	30	213	7–178	3–83
s	60	142	1–128	.7–92
l	28	78	3– 75	4–96

socially acceptable production of the target phoneme – may be present. If the desired response can be located by currently-available testing procedures, it can be reinforced contingently and thus accelerated.

Table V, *Selected Sensory Input Characteristics,* emphasizes a major advantage of building in articulatory therapy. Conventional articulatory therapy has frequently emphasized auditory input. As is indicated in Table V, a subject may receive auditory input either from himself or from another speaker.

The auditory channel has been attractive to the clinician because interpersonal matching and comparison is possible (Van Riper and Irwin, 1964). The somatic channel, on the other hand, provides sensory input only to the speaker. Thus, interpersonal or cross matching of a somatic stimuli in articulation has not been possible.

Yet, if articulation is anything, it is, at least in part, a motor habit. The work of MacNeilage, Rootes and Chase (1967), among others, has indicated that motor habits are monitored primarily by somatic sensations, i.e. proprioceptive-kinesthetic and tactile sensations. To the extent that articulation is a motor habit, the most direct monitoring must be somatic rather than auditory or visual. By virtue of requiring the presence of the desired response, building provides for somatic as well as auditory monitoring. For these and the previously stated reasons, building was selected as

TABLE V

SELECTED SENSORY INPUT CHARACTERISTICS

SENSORY INPUT	*SOURCE–*	
	Other	*Self*
Somatic (Tactile and Proprioceptive-Kinesthetic)	No	Yes
Auditory	Yes	Yes

the primary acceleration technique to be used in the *Paired-Stimuli* procedures.

As will be shown in the next section, *Administration of the Paired-Stimuli Technique,* building can be employed either with a child who has the phoneme in his repertoire or with one who has learned to articulate it acceptably in a specific phonetic environment as a result of training. The essential difference is that in the first situation, the intermittent target behavior (socially acceptable production of the target phoneme) is already available; in the second, it is taught in one (or at most, two) selected phonetic environments.

Linguistics and Learning Theory

It is, of course, misleading to refer to traditional articulatory therapy if by such reference one implies a static concept that has had relatively universal acceptance. But, if one may use the term traditional articulatory therapy as representing historical accumulation, it is probably appropriate to note that much of traditional articulatory therapy has emphasized performance rather than competence. In this connection, certain parallels with learning theory and with linguistics are revealing.

Hull (1943) has emphasized the importance of the consequences of behavior in the learning process. The operant school, of course, is essentially atheoretical. But one implication both from theorists such as Hull and from the basic operant paradigm certainly has been that the behavior that is reinforced is the behavior that is learned. Contingent reinforcement thus became the basic learning technique. And, if one regards performance as synonymous with learning, the strength of the operant position becomes obvious.

Certain theorists such as Guthrie (1934) and Mednick (1964) have made a sharp distinction between learning and performance. If this distinction is made, performance becomes a combination of learning plus motivation. In this framework, then, the important element in learning is contiguity, which is responsible for learning, and the important element in performance is reinforcement, which is responsible for motivation.

Interestingly enough, certain theorists in linguistics are making similar distinctions between what is known and what is done. Traditional or descriptive linguistics has tended to emphasize performance. Generative linguistics has tended to emphasize competence. If this distinction is made, competence is what is known and performance is what is done (Deese, 1970). Performance thus becomes a combination, as in learning theory, of what is known plus motivation.

A distinction should be made, however, between learning theory and linguistics. As noted in Table VI, *Three Approaches to Learning,* a basic tenet in much of learning theory is that learning is common across species. Linguistics, on the other hand, argues that language learning is species specific. Thus, the precise language learned, such as French, German or Ghetto Black, is a function of contiguity, but the ability to learn any oral language is a function of being human.

Present-day speech pathology is beginning to emphasize the distinction between competence and performance. Since speech pathology is concerned with language and not with general human learning, competence in speech pathology currently emphasizes

TABLE VI

THREE APPROACHES TO LEARNING

LEARNING THEORY	*LINGUISTICS*	*SPEECH PATHOLOGY*
Competence Contiguity	Competence Contiguity Species Specific	Competence Contiguity Species Specific Individual Differences
Performance Reinforcement and Punishment	Performance Reinforcement and Punishment	Performance Reinforcement and Punishment Individual Differences

contiguity (the precise language), the faculty of being human and — since speech pathology is a clinical field — individual differences in such attributes as intelligence, neurological integrity, social adjustment and hearing. As in the other fields, performance becomes a combination of competence plus reinforcement and/or punishment. Again, however, in speech pathology the importance of individual differences in basic abilities must be emphasized.

As currently employed, the *Paired-Stimuli Technique* (1) emphasizes performance and does not take systematic cognizance of competence in the sense, for example, of selecting either key words or training words on the basis of linguistic features and (2) except for its self-screening features, minimizes the importance of such individual differences as cleft palate, cerebral palsy or mental retardation. However, nothing in the method precludes the ultimate application of these principles.

ADMINISTRATION OF THE PAIRED-STIMULI TECHNIQUE

Locating Key Words and Training Words

Prior to the initiation of the *Paired-Stimuli* modification procedures, the first target phoneme, a key word or words, and the appropriate number of training words for the phoneme must be determined. In order to locate target phonemes for a subject, any of a variety of articulation tests may be used. Where a large number of children must be evaluated in a short time, screening devices such as the *Triota Screening Battery* (Irwin, 1971b), the *Templin-Darley Tests of Articulation* (1968) or the *Screening Deep Test of Articulation* (McDonald, 1968) may be used to identify children who may require additional evaluation in order to establish their candidacy for articulatory therapy. In Chapter 9, Turton outlines a program of articulatory evaluation which may be used in conjunction with most management programs. After the completion of selected articulatory measures, the sequence in which sounds will be treated must be determined. Irwin (1972), and Turton in the present book, have suggested several criteria that are useful in developing a modification plan.

The first requirement for a suitable target phoneme is that the child misarticulate the phoneme in at least ten words where the phoneme is in either the initial or final position of the words. In the *Paired-Stimuli Technique,* no words are used in training where the target phoneme occurs in the so-called medial position. Thus, for a person who misarticulates the target phoneme. in only the initial or final position of words, ten words must be found where the misarticulated phoneme occurs in the appropriate position. For a person who misarticulates the target phoneme in both the releasing and arresting positions of words, a total of twenty training words must be found, ten where the target phoneme occurs in the initial position and ten with it in the final position.

For use in the *Paired-Stimuli Technique,* a suitable target phoneme is not only one which is misarticulated in some way, but one for which the requisite number of training words can be found. The nature of the misarticulation of any phoneme is considered in developing a sequence of sounds to be modified. It should be pointed out, however, that phonemes which are frequently omitted and/or substituted lend themselves particularly well to the location of the required number of training words.

Training Words. Training words are defined as words in which the target phoneme appears only once, in either the initial or final position, and where the target phoneme is misarticulated in at least two out of three attempts to say words which contain the phoneme when they are presented in groups of ten or more per position (initial or final). The commercially available *Paired-Stimuli Kit* includes pairs of picture sheets for fourteen of the most frequently misarticulated consonant sounds. The first sheet of each pair contains twenty different pictures of words which have the target phoneme in the initial position; the second sheet includes twenty pictures of words with the target phoneme in the final position. Frequently these sheets of pictures can be helpful in locating training words and key words. The child is asked to name each picture while the clinician judges the social acceptability of the child's production of the target phoneme in each word. This procedure is repeated two more times, for a total of three presentations of the twenty pictures. Any word in which the subject misarticulates the target phoneme in at least two repetitions of the twenty words qualifies as a training word. For children who misarticulate the target phoneme in both the initial and final positions of words, a second group of ten training words must be located, with the target phoneme in the appropriate position. These ten words can be sought by using the second sheet of pictures available for the phoneme.

Key Words. Key words can often be located during the process of the child's naming the twenty pictures available for the target phoneme in one position. A key word is defined as one in which the subject produces the target phoneme in a socially acceptable manner; it must have the target phoneme in it only once, in either the initial or the final position. In showing a subject the pictures for the target phoneme in a particular position, it frequently happens that the child produces the target phoneme acceptably in one or more of the words. Any word in which the subject produces the target phoneme acceptably at least two times out of the three presentations is a potential key word. The criterion for the use of any word as a key word is that the target phoneme be produced in a socially acceptable manner *at least nine out of ten times.* Thus, any potential key words obtained from presenting the sheet of pictures three times must be evaluated an additional seven times. Where more than one of the potential key words satisfies the criterion, any one of the words may be used as the key word for the subject. In certain instances, to be discussed later, a second key word may also be sought.

A key word may be taught to the child if one is not found in his repertoire during the search for training words. The procedures recommended for teaching a key word are detailed in *A Manual for the Clinical Utilization of the Paired-Stimuli Technique* (Irwin and Weston, 1971), which is included as part of the *Paired-Stimuli Kit.* The criterion for a taught key word is the same as that for a key word from the child's repertoire: at least nine out of ten socially acceptable productions of the target phoneme, within the context of words.

Training Procedures

Training Strings. When all of the training words for a particular phoneme have been located from the picture sheets, the pictures are peeled off the adhesive-backed picture sheet and placed on the *Paired-Stimuli Sheet* in the appropriate spaces. The key word is placed in the center of the sheet. When the clinician has located a key word and training words appropriate to the target phoneme and prepared the *Paired-Stimuli Sheet,* the training procedures may be initiated. These involve the subject's alternately naming the key word and each of ten training words for the target phoneme in a particular position. During the pairing procedure, the child is given a tangible reinforcer, such as a poker chip, for every socially acceptable production of the target phoneme, whether it be in the key word or in a training word, irrespective of the subject's articulation of the other phonemes in the words. These tokens are redeemable at the end of each therapy period for back-up reinforcers, such as toys, candy or money. The contingent pairing of the key word with each of the ten training words in one position constitutes a training string. Three training strings must be completed during each training session. The training strings afford the subject an opportunity to earn tokens for producing the target phoneme in a socially acceptable manner. Early in training, a child may earn few, if any, tokens for the production of the target phoneme in training words because they are, by definition, phonetic environments in which he does not produce the target phoneme acceptably. However, he should produce the target phoneme in the key word acceptably at least nine out of ten times in each string. Otherwise, the key word is regarded as unstable and training must be temporarily discontinued, so that the key word may be brought to criterion again. With the continued contingent pairing of the key word and each training word, the child's correct production of the target phoneme in the key word begins to generalize to the training words, which are then also reinforced with tokens. Socially acceptable production of the target phoneme in the training words under contingent reinforcement is a sub-goal of the procedures; the desired terminal behavior is a socially acceptable production of the target phoneme in the training words and in spontaneous speech without tangible reinforcement. Therefore, probes are administered prior to and following each group of three training strings.

Probes. Probes are designed to measure the extent to which a subject produces the target phoneme acceptably in the key word and in all twenty training words (ten words for each of two positions — initial and final) under conditions of no reinforcement. In the probe which precedes each training session (pre-probe), the subject is asked to name the key word and each of the twenty training words once. The clinician records the number of socially acceptable productions of the target phoneme in the 21 words — 22 in cases where two key words are employed — but gives the client no reinforcement following productions deemed socially acceptable. The format for the probe which follows the third training string for each training session (post-probe) is identical with the pre-probe. The post-probe is especially important because the subject's performance dictates when training on the target phoneme in a particular position or training on an entire phoneme may be terminated.

Criterion. Criterion is defined as the socially acceptable production of at least eight of the ten training words for a particular position on two successive post-probes. Though these post-probes must be successive, they need not occur on the same day, i.e. if a subject produces the target phoneme socially acceptably in eight or more of the ten training words on the final post-probe of a particular day and duplicates this performance on the first post-probe of the next therapy day, criterion has been reached. Despite the fact that all twenty training words are evaluated during probes, criterion is defined only in terms of the position currently being trained. The purpose of evaluating the untrained words is to determine whether any generalization to them occurs as a result of training on the first ten words; when the second ten words are being trained, the retention of acceptable production of the target phoneme in the previously-trained words is measured by the probe.

When criterion is reached on the first position trained, the training words with the target phoneme in the opposite position of the word must be taught to criterion. When two positions are trained for a phoneme, criterion must be met twice, once for each position. Where only one position has been trained for a phoneme, the next phoneme can be started when the single position for the phoneme has been trained to criterion.

Intervention Designs. In order to provide flexibility in use of the training procedures, six *Intervention Designs* have been described (Irwin and Weston, 1971). The factors which vary in the designs concern (1) whether the key word is from the subject's repertoire or is taught, (2) whether one or two key words are used and (3) the position of the target phoneme in the key word(s). See Table VIII, *Intervention Designs,* which displays the six designs.

Summary of Procedures. In summary, the *Paired-Stimuli* articulatory modification procedures are based on the assumption that a target phoneme produced in a word in a socially acceptable manner can be generalized from that phonetic environment to a variety of other word contexts, through a behavior modification program which emphasizes building procedures. A continuous reinforcement schedule is applied to the socially acceptable production of the target phoneme in any word during a pairing procedure. Criterion for terminating training on a particular position is the socially acceptable production of the target phoneme in at least eight out of ten training words in a particular position over two successive post-probes. In cases where both positions are trained, double criterion is necessary before proceeding to the next target phoneme.

Intra-Session and Inter-Session Measures of Progress

Intra-session and inter-session progress, as discussed in Chapter 9, are carefully assessed as part of the *Paired-Stimuli* training program. During the contingent pairing procedure, judgments are made of the social acceptability of the target phoneme in each key word and each training word, so that changes within the therapy period can be evaluated. Post-probes serve the purpose of assessing progress both within and across therapy periods and determine the point at which a different position of the target phoneme may be trained or a new target phoneme begun. Inter-session progress is evaluated by pre-probes, which are administered prior to the presentation of the training stimuli for each training session. As noted earlier, several training sessions may be held during any one therapy period, each of which normally requires a pre-probe. However, it is permissible for a pre-probe to be given only at the beginning of a therapy period, whereas in current use a post-probe must follow each group of three training strings. The latter requirement is based on the possibility of a subject's reaching criterion within a therapy period, which, in fact, often occurs.

Measures of Rate of Acquisition

The procedures permit the precise recording of progress, which may be used for comparisons within a single child across phonemes or across children on the same phoneme. The rate of improvement is indicated by: (1) total minutes to criterion (typically, double criterion) and (2) number of training sessions to criterion. The speed with which a phoneme can be trained to double criterion is measured by totaling the number of minutes spent in each training session. The number of training sessions to double criterion is related to the number of minutes required to reach this point. However, because the number of minutes required for each training session may vary somewhat, the total number of sessions required to reach criterion may be useful to the clinician in planning future therapy schedules, with allowance made for some variation among children. The recording of all measures of progress as a result of training is simplified by use of forms available in the *Paired-Stimuli Kit.*

Assessment of Generalization

Both formal and informal tests of generalization of training may be made at various points in the training process. Scores on articulation measures given prior to therapy may be repeated and compared during therapy and at its completion for any particular phoneme or group of phonemes. Repeated measurements provide evidence not only of the effect of the modification procedures upon a target phoneme, but certain tests may reveal the extent to which training has affected phonetically similar sounds. For example, the *Screening Deep Test of Articulation* (McDonald, 1968) has been used prior to training, at the time double criterion is reached and two weeks after achieving double criterion. These administrations are designed to indicate baseline, improvement in production of the target phoneme and any generalization to other sounds sampled on the test and the extent to which any improvement as a result of training has been maintained without reinforcement, respectively.

Conversational samples of speech may also be taken at various points in order to assess the extent to which phoneme training affects usage of the sound in spontaneous speech. A schedule of pre-intervention, post-intervention and retention is also useful in this context.

INTERVENTION DATA

Data from a pilot study of the *Paired-Stimuli Technique* will be presented under three headings: *Procedural Variables, Criterion Measures* and *Generalization/Retention Measures.* Although the *Paired-Stimuli Technique* has been used in a variety of environments, the intervention data reported here are based exclusively on therapy done with 126 children, of whom 97 were enrolled in the DeSoto County, Mississippi Schools and 29 in the Osceola, Arkansas School District during the 1970-71 school year. Because of the unavailability of certain data, the sample size varies sbmewhat for some of the variables. Table VII, *Number of Children for Whom Intervention Data Are Reported by Type of Data and by Collection Interval,* gives the sample size for each variable. All data reported pertain only to the first target phoneme trained for each child. The data have been restricted in this fashion primarily because this was the largest single sample for which the procedures were sufficiently controlled to permit meaningful summation and analysis. Moreover, inasmuch as these data were obtained from school children, the results should be widely applicable.

Procedural Variables

At our present state of information concerning the effectiveness of the *Paired-Stimuli Technique,* the major procedural variables undoubtedly relate to the type of *Intervention Design* employed. As noted earlier, six *Intervention Designs* have been devised for

TABLE VII

NUMBER OF CHILDREN FOR WHOM INTERVENTION DATA
ARE REPORTED BY TYPE OF DATA AND BY COLLECTION
INTERVAL

DATA COLLECTION INTERVAL (RE: 1ST TARGET PHONEME)	CRITERION FOR FIRST, SECOND AND BOTH TARGET PHONEME POSITIONS				SCREENING DEEP TEST		H-SCALE RATING ON 3-MINUTE CONVERSATIONS
	TIME IN MINUTES	NO. OF SESSIONS	SLOPE	POST-PROBE VALUES	TARGET PHONEME VALUES	8 OTHER PHONEME VALUES	
Pre-Intervention	0	0	0	126	126	126	126
Post-Intervention	126	114	114	97	97	97	97
Post-Intervention + 2 Weeks	0	0	0	126	126	126	126

flexibility in use of the *Paired-Stimuli Technique.* These designs are depicted in Table VIII, *Intervention Designs.* Each design is determined on the basis of (1) whether the key word is taught or from the child's repertoire, (2) whether one or two key words are used and (3) the position of the target phoneme in the key word. The first two *Intervention Designs* require two key words, where the first key word has its target phoneme in the same position as that of the training words with which it will be paired during training strings (such as final position for both the key word and the training words). The second key word has the target phoneme in the opposite position, as do the ten training words with which it will be paired (initial position for key word and initial position for training words).

Each of the four remaining *Intervention Designs* requires only one key word. In *Intervention Designs* 3 and 4, the target phoneme occurs in the final position of the key word. In *Intervention Designs* 5 and 6, the target phoneme always occurs in the initial position of the key word. In these four designs the same key word is used to train both positions of the target phoneme, i.e. position of the target phoneme in the key word is not a direct function of the position of the target phoneme in the training words.

Other procedural variables include sex, race and age of each subject, clinician and target phoneme. Because of the relatively small sample of subjects (126) involved, it was impossible to study these additional variables by *Intervention Design.* Consequently,

TABLE VIII

INTERVENTION DESIGNS

KEY WORD POSITION	*KEY WORD REPERTOIRE*	*KEY WORD TAUGHT*
Key Words, Initial and Final	1	2
Key Word, Final	3	4
Key Word, Initial	5	6

only sex, race and age data for the entire population will be presented.

Several potentially important procedural variables are: phoneme, error type, position in the word, phonetic environment and sequence in training order of the target phoneme (that is, whether it is the first, second or subsequent phoneme trained). Again, because of limitations of numbers, it was impossible to study these variables. Thus, all data are based on the first phoneme trained and are reported without reference to the specific phoneme involved or its phonetic environment.

As will be discussed in the final section of this chapter, certain other procedural variables can and should be investigated. The listing presented here should not be regarded as definitive but simply as a list of the variables which have been studied to date.

Criterion Measures

Immediate success is defined as reaching double criterion, that is, eight or more socially acceptable productions of the target phoneme on two successive post-probes for each position trained (initial and final). Because criterion is fixed, variation in subject performance appears in factors such as the time required to reach criterion, the number of training sessions (or post-probes), the values (scores) at each post-probe and a computed value, the slope of the acquisition curve. In this condensed report, because intervention time is the crucial element in a practical situation, time has been used as the criterion variable against which the procedural variables can be evaluated.

Intervention Design. Table IX, *Time in Minutes for 126 Children to Reach Double Criterion by Intervention Design,* gives the relevant data. The means and ranges shown suggest that each of the *Intervention Designs* is roughly equivalent in its efficiency, although approximately 20 minutes must be added when a key word is taught if the clinician has first sought to locate a key word in the child's repertoire unsuccessfully. At the moment, the mean of 46 minutes for *Intervention Design* 2 may be an artifact of the teaching procedures employed. Although the data do not permit rigorous substantiation of this statement, there is reason to believe

TABLE IX

TIME IN MINUTES FOR 126 CHILDREN TO REACH
DOUBLE CRITERION BY INTERVENTION DESIGN

			INTERVENTION DESIGN					
			(1) F/I–R	(2) F/I–T	(3) F–R	(4) F–T	(5) I–R	(6) I–T
N		126	9	11	26	59	7	14
Minutes	Mean	79	84	46	85	76	81	94
	Range	25-245	50-135	25-70	30-185	25-245	25-230	30-160

that the key word was *over-taught* to the children assigned to this design, which may account for its being noticeably shorter. Procedures presently employed control for this possibility.

On the basis of these pilot data, taking into account the possibility of over-teaching the key word in *Intervention Design 2*, the tentative conclusion is that each of the *Intervention Designs* is clinically practicable. It is to be hoped that further data will support this conclusion, as this finding would allow great flexibility to the clinician.

Sex, Race, and Age of Subjects. In Table X, *Time in Minutes for 126 Children to Reach Double Criterion by Sex, Race and Age*, shows that on the average, female subjects achieved double criterion 15 minutes faster than did boys. By inspection, there is no significant difference between black children and white children in terms of the time required to reach double criterion. The mean time for the children 8.5 years and younger was 83 minutes; for those aged 9 and older, 73 minutes. These pilot figures suggest that the technique is relatively independent of age. This tentative finding may be of importance to clinicians who work with older children.

Clinician. Sixteen clinicians participated in this study. Because some of them worked with as few as two children, a formal

TABLE X

TIME IN MINUTES FOR 126 CHILDREN TO REACH
DOUBLE CRITERION BY SEX, RACE AND AGE

		N	*MEAN*	*RANGE*
Sex	Male	74	85	25-230
	Female	52	70	25-245
Race	Black	61	79	30-245
	White	64	78	25-185
Age	8.5 Years and Under	68	83	25-245
	9.0 Years and Older	58	73	25-230

analysis of the data is not presented. It should be noted, however, that a wide range in mean time to criterion by clinician was observed. For example, one clinician averaged 46 minutes with each of her clients to bring them to double criterion, while another clinician averaged 119 minutes. 'If we assume that the problems of their clients were of comparable difficulty, these figures strongly suggest wide individual differences in the rate with which clinicians bring children to criterion. On the basis of the pilot study, the data provide us neither with clues as to the bases for any such differences nor to any possible long-range effects of these differences in mean training times. Therefore, it can only be said that some clinicians bring children to criterion more rapidly than do others.

Generalization/Retention Measures

Two measures will be reviewed in this section: measures on *A Screening Deep Test of Articulation* (McDonald, 1968) and ratings on a communicative-handicappingness scale. Tape-recordings of conversational speech were made for the purpose of computing percentages of acceptable usage of the target phoneme in spontaneous speech prior to intervention, at the time double criterion was reached and two weeks after having reached double criterion. However, poor quality of the tape recordings did not permit successful judgments.

Measures Based on A Screening Deep Test of Articulation. On the day on which therapy was initiated (or the day before such therapy was begun, in certain instances) each subject was administered *A Screening Deep Test of Articulation* (McDonald, 1968). The number of acceptable productions of each of the nine phonemes tested was recorded. In each case, one of these nine phonemes constituted the target phoneme. On the day criterion was reached for the second position trained (or on the first therapy day following the reaching of double criterion), the *Screening Deep Test* was again administered. Finally, two weeks after reaching double criterion, the McDonald test was given again.

For 29 of the children, the *Screening Deep Test* was not administered at the time double criterion was reached. Table XI, *Screening Deep Test* (McDonald) *by Data Collection Interval and Phoneme Category,* summarizes the data. The significant findings are that (1) the percent of acceptable productions of the target phoneme increased from the pre-intervention to the post-intervention period and was maintained in the measure taken two weeks later and (2) the percentage of acceptable articulation of the other eight phonemes did not vary materially at any of the three testing periods. This finding suggests that the *Paired-Stimuli Technique* has minimal side effects — either good or bad — on phonemes other than the target phoneme.

Communicative Handicappingness Scale Measures. On the day on which therapy was begun (or on the day before therapy was initiated), a three-minute conversation between the clinician and the subject was recorded on audio tape. Immediately after the conversation, the clinician rated the child's speech on the *Communicative Handicappingness Scale.* Values on this scale ranged from 0 to 1000. A scale value of 100 represented the level at which clinical speech intervention was judged as just necessary;

TABLE XI

SCREENING DEEP TEST (McDONALD) BY DATA
COLLECTION INTERVAL AND PHONEME CATEGORY

DATA COLLECTION INTERVAL (RE: 1ST TARGET PHONEME)	MEAN: TARGET PHONEME		MEAN: 8 OTHER PHONEMES	
	97 Children	126* Children	97 Children	126 Children
Pre-Intervention	2.05	1.99	8.57	6.98
Post-Intervention	6.96	Not Available	8.82	Not Available
Post-Intervention + 2 Weeks	6.61	6.40	9.00	7.02

*The sample of 126 includes the sample of 97.

0 represented speech which constituted no handicap; and 1000 represented speech which was maximally handicapping. Table XII, *Mean Communicative Handicappingness Ratings by Data Collection Intervals,* presents these data. Note that the ratings decrease following intervention and two weeks after double criterion has been reached. That the final rating does not become less than 100 is not surprising; most of these children had multiple articulatory deviations, and these values were obtained only on the first phoneme trained.

Variables Which May Be Significantly Related to Treatment Outcome. The current procedures employed in the *Paired-Stimuli Technique* reflect decisions made as a result of preliminary investigations aimed at developing a methodology which was both economical of clinical time and which produced satisfactory results. For example, the number of training words per position was set at ten in early use of the technique (Weston, 1969) and has

TABLE XII

MEAN COMMUNICATIVE HANDICAPPINGNESS RATINGS
BY DATA COLLECTION INTERVALS

DATA COLLECTION INTERVAL (RE: 1ST TARGET PHONEME)	MEAN COMMUNICATIVE HANDICAPPINGNESS RATINGS	
	97 Children	126* Children
Pre-Intervention	157	149
Post-Intervention	125	Not Available
Post-Intervention + 2 Weeks	112	113

*The sample of 126 includes the sample of 97.

been maintained so that its efficiency could be evaluated on large numbers of children. However, the basic value of any technique designed to modify specific behaviors rests upon the identification and exploration of variables which appear pertinent to its assumptions and its most efficient use. A number of potentially significant variables are indicated below, certain of which are currently under investigation. The designations are arbitrary; these variables may interact with one another in a variety of ways in specific cases.

Nature and Consistency of Misarticulation

The rate of success in use of the *Paired-Stimuli Technique* may be related to the nature and consistency of misarticulated target phonemes. As Turton has pointed out in Chapter 9, certain phonological features may be represented in a number of misarticulated phonemes. Due recognition of such a possibility in the overall plan of modification might increase the efficiency of management programs. With regard to the *Paired-Stimuli Technique,* it may be that explicit consideration of cross-phoneme features is more efficient than considering phonemes for modification on the basis of norms of acquisition, the latter being the current practice.

The rate of acquisition of a phoneme may also be related to variables such as the age of the subject and his predominant error pattern for a particular phoneme. For example, a pre-school-age child who primarily omits a phoneme may acquire acceptable production of the sound at a different, though not necessarily slower, rate from that of a second-grader or third-grader who tends to substitute another phoneme for the target sound. Elbert (1971) suggested that for children aged six and older, who display primarily substitution or distortion errors on the /s/ or /r/ phonemes, the type of misarticulation does not change as a result of therapy, although the rate of correct production does. The generality of this finding might be profitably explored using the *Paired-Stimuli Technique,* on the assumption that lack of change in error type found in Elbert's study might have been a function of the heterogeneity of intervention procedures used by her clinicians.

Number of Training Words

The number of training words necessary to effect a desired level of carry-over to spontaneous speech should be investigated. Acceptable generalization to spontaneous speech may require varying numbers of training words for different children or for different phonemes, depending on factors such as the ages of the children and the nature and consistency of their misarticulation patterns. There may be a critical range of training words necessary to produce the desired level of carry-over to spontaneous speech which is related to certain phonetic profiles or patterns of misarticulation.

Schedules of Reinforcement

Currently, all socially acceptable productions of the target phoneme are consequated on a continuous reinforcement schedule (FRI) during training strings. It is premature to assume that the present schedule of reinforcement is the most efficient schedule for most children, or that a different single schedule can be evolved which is efficient for a majority of children on this program. It may be that, ultimately, individualized schedules of reinforcement will be the answer.

Phonetic Environments

The phonetic environments of key words and/or training words may be related to rate of acquisition and carry-over. Whether the immediate phonetic environment of the key word (the phoneme which precedes or follows the target phoneme) and that of the training words should be similar is a question of interest. For example, where /s/ is the target phoneme and *stove* is a key word from the subject's repertoire, should the training words also be presented in an sC or Cs environment (where s represents the target phoneme and C represents any consonant) for most rapid acquisition? Implicit in this question is also that of whether training words which have a specific phonetic environment (target phoneme preceded or followed by a vowel or diphthong versus the target phoneme preceded or followed by a consonant) generalize across phonetic environments satisfactorily in conversational speech. Obviously, information regarding this issue would be particularly helpful in situations where a key word cannot be found in the child's repertoire and must, therefore, be taught.

Familiarity of Training Words

Does the rate of phoneme acquisition and carry-over to spontaneous speech depend upon a subject's familiarity with the training words? Despite the presentation of the target phoneme within the context of a meaningful unit, it might be argued that words unfamiliar to the subject are akin to nonsense syllables. If the assumption is made that linguistic meaningfulness is important to acquisition and carry-over, the words represented by the picture stimuli assume some importance. The training words available in the *Paired-Stimuli Kit* were constructed with primary concern for their picturability, although an effort was made to include pictures of objects familiar to many young children. These stimuli pictures were regarded as neither an articulation test nor as a vocabulary test. For example, it is permissible to name a picture for a child if he does not recognize it and to include such a picture in the training procedures.

Linguistic Aspects of the Stimuli

Because nouns lend themselves to pictorial representation more readily than do other linguistic units, most of the picture stimuli from the *Paired-Stimuli Kit* are of this type. Related to the notion of familiarity, discussed above, is the concept of linguistic appropriateness. Despite the fact that nouns are the primary constituent of the language of very young children, it may be that particular target phonemes occur in linguistic units such as verbs, adverbs, pronouns or adjectives more frequently in the speech of older subjects. Therefore, it might be that carry-over would be greater, or more rapid, if certain of these units were represented in the stimuli, rather than nouns. Obviously a clinician is free to choose whatever stimulus materials he considers most appropriate; the commercially available stimulus pictures are provided primarily as a reasonable source of key words and training words. However, the relationship between the picture stimuli and carry-over, versus other types of stimuli (different pictures, graphemes, etc.) and their carry-over, has not been demonstrated at this point.

Interference Factors

In current practice, a subject is given a two-week respite from therapy at the time he reaches double criterion on a phoneme. At the end of this time, the currently used generalization/retention measures are made. These measures are *A Screening Deep Test of*

Articulation (McDonald, 1968) and a tape-recording of spontaneous speech. The primary purpose of this break from therapy was to reduce the likelihood of the first sound's interfering with training on the next phoneme and to allow for stabilization of progress on the first trained sound. The two-week hiatus was considered ample for these purposes.

It is clear that the validity of the assumptions underlying the two-week break from therapy needs to be tested. The precaution regarding possible interference by initiating training on a new phoneme close to the completion of training on the previous one may be unnecessary. If this proves to be the case, then the time span required for remediation of several phonemes can be reduced significantly.

Furthermore, in keeping with Turton's discussion in Chapter 9, it may be that if training is initiated on a second sound soon after termination of training on the first and the two phonemes are similar in their distinctive features, facilitation of either or both of the sounds might result.

REFERENCES

Aronson, A.: Speech pathology and symptom therapy in the interdisciplinary treatment of psychogenic aphonia. J Speech Hear Disord, 34:321-341, 1969.

Azrin, N. H., and Holz, W. C.: Punishment. In W. K. Honig (Ed.): Operant Behavior: Areas of Research and Application. New York, Appleton-Century-Crofts, Inc., 1966.

Birnbrauer, J. S., Wolf, M. M., Kidder, J. D., and Teague, C. E.: Classroom behavior of retarded pupils with token reinforcement. J Exp Child Psychol, 2:219-235, 1965.

Brookshire, R. H.: Speech pathology and the experimental analysis of behavior. J Speech Hear Disord, 32:215-227, 1967.

Davis, H., and Silverman, R.: Hearing and Deafness, 3rd ed. New York, Holt, Rinehart and Winston, 1970.

Deese, J.: Psycholinguistics. Boston, Allyn and Bacon, Inc., 1970.

Elbert, M.: The effects of therapy on distortion, substitution and omission errors. Paper presented at the 1971 Convention of the American Speech and Hearing Association, Chicago.

Eysenck, H. J.: Learning theory and behavior therapy. In H. J. Eysenck (Ed.) Behavior Therapy and the Neuroses. New York, Pergamon Press, 1960.

Griffith, F. A.: The effects of positive reinforcement and two ratios of token gain to token loss upon imitative speech responses. Paper presented at the 1971 Convention of the American Speech and Hearing Association, Chicago.

Guthrie, E. R.: Reward and punishment. Psychol Rev, 41:450-460, 1934.

Harlow, H. F.: The effects of social isolation upon the intellectual capabilities of the rhesus monkey. Association Luncheon Address, 43rd Annual Convention, American Speech and Hearing Association, 1967, Chicago.

Hull, C. L.: Principles of Behavior. New York, Appleton, 1943.

Irwin, J. V.: Symptom substitution? Acta Symbolica, 2:19-21, 1971.

Irwin, J. V.: Computer application in speech pathology. Short Course: 47th Annual Convention, American Speech and Hearing Association, 1971, Chicago.

Irwin, J. V.: Introduction to Communicative Disorders. Boston, Allyn and Bacon, Inc., in preparation.

Irwin, J. V.: Articulation. In A. J. Weston (Ed.) Communicative Disorders: An Appraisal. Springfield, Thomas, 1972.

Irwin, J. V., and Weston, A. J.: A Manual for the Clinical Utilization of the Paired-Stimuli Technique. Memphis; National Educator Services, Inc., 1971.

Kohler, W.: The Mentality of Apes. New York; Harcourt, Brace, 1925.

Logan, F. A., and Wagner, A. R.: Reward and Punishment. Boston; Allyn and Bacon, Inc., 1966.

MacNeilage, P. F., Rootes, T. P., and Chase, R. A.: Speech production and perception in a patient with severe impairment of somesthetic perception and motor control. J Speech Hear Res, 10:449-467, 1967.

McDonald, E. T.: A Deep Test of Articulation. Pittsburgh; Stanwix House, Inc., 1964.

McDonald, E. T.: A Screening Deep Test of Articulation. Pittsburgh, Stanwix House, Inc., 1968.

McReynolds, L. V., and Huston, K.: Token loss in speech imitation training. J Speech Hear Disord, 36:486-495, 1971.

Mednick, S. A.: Learning. Englewood Cliffs, Prentice-Hall, Inc., 1964.

Minifie, F., Burkhart, M., and Wentland, T.: Deep articulation testing and the public schools. J Wisc Speech Hear, 4:1-10, 1966.

Moses, P. J.: The Voice of Neurosis. New York, Grune and Stratton, 1954.

Murphy, A. T.: Stuttering, behavior modification and the person. Conditioning in Stuttering Therapy. Memphis, Speech Foundation of America, 1970.

Newby, H. A.: Audiology, 2nd Ed. New York, Appleton-Century-Crofts, Inc., 1964.

O'Neill, J. J., and Oyer, H. J.: Applied Audiometry. New York, Dodd, Mead and Co., 1966.

Perkins, W. H.: The challenge of functional disorders of voice. In L. E. Travis (Ed.) Handbook of Speech Pathology. New York, Appleton-Century-Crofts, Inc., 1957.

Rousey, C. L., and Moriarty, A. E.: Diagnostic Implications of Speech Sounds. Springfield, Thomas, 1965.

Sajwaj, T. E.: Some parameters of point loss. Unpublished doctoral dissertation, University of Kansas, 1969.

Sataloff, J.: Hearing Loss. Philadelphia, J. B. Lippincott Co., 1966.

Skinner, B. F.: Walden Two. New York, MacMillan, 1948.

Skinner, B. F.: Are theories of learning necessary? Psychol Rev, 57:193-216, 1950.

Skinner, B. F.: Science and Human Behavior. New York, MacMillan, 1953.

Sloane, H. N., Jr., and MacAulay, B. D.: Operant Procedures in Remedial Speech and Language Training. Boston, Houghton Mifflin Company, 1968.

Solomon, R. L.: Punishment. Am Psychol, 19:239-253, 1964.

Spence, K. W.: Theoretical interpretations of learning. In S. S. Stevens (ed.) Handbook of Experimental Psychology. New York, John Wiley and Sons, 1951.

Templin, M. C., and Darley, F. L.: The Templin-Darley Tests of Articulation. Iowa City, Bureau of Educational Research and Service, Extension Division, State University of Iowa, 1968.

Thorndike, E. L.: Animal Intelligence. New York, MacMillan, 1911.

Thorndike, E. L.: Educational Psychology, vol. II. The Psychology of Learning. New York, Teachers College, Columbia University, 1913.

Thorndike, E. L.: Human Learning. New York, MacMillan, 1931.

Van Riper, C.: Symptomatic therapy for stuttering. In L. E. Travis (Ed.) Handbook of Speech Pathology. New York, Appleton-Century-Crofts, Inc., 1957.

Van Riper, C., and Irwin, J. V.: Voice and Articulation. Englewood Cliffs, Prentice-Hall, Inc., 1964.

Weiner, H.: Response cost of fixed-ratio performance. J Exp Anal Behav, 7:79-81, 1964.

Weston, A. J.: The use of paired-stimuli in the modification of articulation. Doctoral dissertation, University of Kansas, 1969.

Weston, A. J., and Irwin, J. V.: Use of paired-stimuli in modification of articulation. Percept Mot Skills, 32:947-957, 1971.

CHAPTER IX

DIAGNOSTIC IMPLICATIONS OF ARTICULATION TESTING

LAWRENCE J. TURTON

THE purpose of this chapter is to evaluate the role of articulation tests in the total therapy process and to discuss a broader concept of articulation testing. Three topics will receive particular attention:

(1) Behavioral Evaluation of Articulation Skills
(2) Scoring and Analyzing Articulation Tests
(3) The Process of Generalization

These three topics were selected because they relate to the clinical hypothesis upon which this chapter is based: the division of clinical activities of speech pathology into diagnostic and therapy tasks is a false dichotomy. When we accept a child into a therapy program, we are entering into a contractual relationship that requires us to provide the most efficient and complete service possible. One critical aspect of this service is to have available a complete picture of a child's articulation profile at all times. Clinical researchers have now developed measuring devices or procedures that permit the speech clinician to maintain relatively accurate records of a child's progress.

BEHAVIORAL EVALUATION OF ARTICULATION SKILLS

Testing During Initial Sessions

Texts of diagnostic procedures in speech pathology (Johnson, Darley and Spriestersbach, 1963; Darley, 1964) instruct the

195

clinician to rule out possible contributing or etiological variables in the articulatory problem by screening the child for a hearing loss, intellectual deficits, emotional problems or social problems. Consequently, we have established procedures which we follow in a *diagnostic* session in addition to administering the speech and language tests. Quite often, the assignment of a diagnostic label (e.g. *functional articulation problem*) signals the termination of all testing activity until the child is to be dismissed from therapy either for a clinical vacation or because therapy is no longer needed. Measures of progress are frequently comprised of subjective evaluations on the part of the clinician regarding the articulation status of the child.

For the term *diagnosis,* perhaps we should substitute the term *behavioral evaluation.* Essentially, we should be obtaining a continuous description of the articulation status of the child. A behavioral evaluation of the articulation skills of a child should provide the clinician with a description of the many variables that constitute the phonological system and contribute to the therapy program. The behavioral description should be constantly updated throughout the therapy program. In terms of procedures, a behavioral evaluation views the *diagnostic* session as the first therapy session in which a preliminary baseline of articulation behavior is obtained and a judgement is made as to which sound(s) will receive initial emphasis in subsequent sessions. Furthermore, preliminary information should be obtained from the child which will facilitate the process of deciding on the form of therapy (i.e. *ear-training* or *phonetic placement*) and the frequency of therapy. On the basis of information gathered in this session, the types of intra- and inter-session measures should be tentatively selected.

The first evaluation session should include as a minimum the following types of articulation tests: (1) spontaneous picture tests, (2) imitative tests, (3) tests for misarticulations in specific phonetic contexts, (4) stimulability testing and (5) auditory discrimination testing. This testing battery can be easily assembled by any clinician from readily available commercial tests or by constructing specific tests for individual children. Many clinicians have extensive experience with these tests; however, not all five types of tests are always used in the evaluation session.

Despite the discussion in the literature concerning the differences between spontaneous and imitative testing, we should incorporate both modes of testing into the evaluation process. Each form of testing provides a slightly different picture of the articulation skills of the child. The two modes of assessing articulation behavior should be viewed as methods for providing supportive evidence for clinical decisions and not as mutually exclusive forms of testing.

There have also been recent attempts in the literature to eliminate three-position (initial, medial, final) word testing in articulation appraisals. Relying almost solely upon physiologically-oriented theoretical constructs, McDonald (1964) and others have suggested that three-item testing be relegated to a minor role when testing articulation behavior. On the other hand, there is sufficient evidence to suggest that we need to retain all forms of word positions as well as phonetic context testing. All forms of articulation behavior are controlled by the phonological rules of the language and must be accounted for in the articulation assessment. Indeed, the definite possibility exists that the physiological constructs often mentioned by McDonald are *passive* forms of behavior that conform to or interact with the *active* linguistic rules of the phonological patterns of the culture. The rejection of either three-item testing or phonetic context testing could be a critical clinical mistake by our profession. As with the difference between spontaneous and imitative forms of testing, three-item testing and phonetic context testing are best viewed as two portions of a complete articulation battery.

In addition to three-item testing and phonetic context testing, we should also consider assessing sound productions in linguistic units of varying length, hereafter referred to as *linguistic context* testing. Since we have built a tradition of performing articulation therapy according to a sequence of sound-in-isolation, nonsense syllables, words, phrases, sentences and conversational speech, we need baseline information on the level of linguistic context at which a child has the most difficulty. The skill of production at the isolation and nonsense syllable level can be easily determined as one aspect of the analysis of the stimulability testing or special consideration can be given to them during the testing session.

Word production (both spontaneously and imitatively) is also an accepted part of present testing procedures. Higher level linguistic contexts, however, have only recently been incorporated into tests. The *Goldman-Fristoe Test of Articulation* (Goldman and Fristoe, 1969) and a special 223-item test developed by Shelton and his associates (Elbert, Shelton and Ardnt, 1967; Shelton, Elbert and Ardnt, 1967) for research purposes have the sentence/ conversation levels incorporated into them. In the former test, the *Words-in-Conversation* section is considered a form of spontaneous testing. However, the manner of eliciting the responses reduces the section to a form of *delayed-imitation* testing. It is, nonetheless, a good example of a successful, innovative test form. The Shelton test has only an imitation section for phrases and sentences. Table I presents selected items and sections of the 223-item test as modified by Park (1968). Park changed some of the items depicted in the spontaneous section and arranged the sounds randomly rather than by developmental levels to avoid an age bias during testing.

Stimulability testing for prognostic purposes has received only limited interest by our profession. The studies by Carter and Buck (1958) and Farquahar (1961) comprise the major works in this area. Sommers *et al.* (1967) have evaluated the importance of degrees of stimulability as they relate to success in therapy. Goldman and Fristoe (1969) have included a stimulability section in their test which measures performance on this task through the phrase level of linguistic context.

Although the total clinical value of stimulability has yet to be tested and demonstrated, sufficient evidence exists to justify its inclusion in the test battery. At least for first-grade children (Carter and Buck, 1958), this type of testing has been shown to have predictive value. Stimulability testing also provides some information regarding the phonetic skills of a child which is important for planning therapy. The child who does not produce a sound under spontaneous testing, but does under imitative and/or stimulability testing, evidences ability to manipulate the articulators to produce the sound, even though he is not using the sound systematically. Stimulability and imitative testing may reflect

TABLE I

SELECTED FRICATIVE AND AFFRICATE ITEMS
FROM THE 223–ITEM ARTICULATION TEST

Phonemes	Spontaneous Words	Imitated Words	Isolation	Imitated Phrases
ʃ	shoe dishes fish	ship ocean wish	ʃ	He lost his shirt. The washer is broken. Is that a new brush?
θ	thread toothbrush teeth	thumb bathtub with	θ	I have thirty cents. When is your birthday? I took a bath.
s	sun bicycle house	soup beside bus	s	Where is my suit? His father is a policeman. He caught a mouse.
z	zebra scissors eggs	zipper daisy nose	z	We went to the zoo. Are you busy? Watch out for bees!
f	five elephant giraffe	fun coffee leaf	f	My feet are cold. Practice safety. Buy me a loaf.
v	valentine shovel glove	voice over stove	v	What a pretty vase! We swam in the river. Where is my cave?
ð	feather	this mother smooth	ð	I like them. Is that your father? At night they bathe.
ʒ	television garage	measure rouge	ʒ	It's a pleasure to meet you. We saw a mirage.
tʃ	chair matches witch	chain pitcher watch	tʃ	Did you see the chipmunk? Mother went to the butcher. Where is your church?
dʒ	jump soldier cage	jar angel bridge	dʒ	Do you like jelly? He played soldier. She bought cabbage.

phonetic skills whereas spontaneous testing may reflect phonemic* skills. Thus, the different results obtained under the two modes of testing may be partially explained because they tap different phonological skills.

Auditory discrimination testing has had an uneven (though time-honored) history in our profession. Despite several attempts to develop effective clinical tests, our profession has not been able to agree upon the type or format of auditory discrimination tests. The emphasis upon auditory-oriented therapy programs, however, dictates that we measure this skill at some point in the course of the evaluation. An intelligent decision to utilize an auditory approach to therapy for a child can best be made with evidence that the child has a deficiency in discrimination.

Originally, auditory discrimination tests attempted to measure a general deficit in discrimination. Gradually the profession has been moving to the position that auditory discrimination deficits, when present, are related to the sounds which are in error. The deficits appear to be not general, but phoneme-bound, i.e. specific. Still unanswered, however, is the broader question of the interaction between identifiable auditory discrimination errors and misarticulations. Whether one causes the other or whether there is some deficient system that depresses both auditory discrimination and articulation skills remains to be answered by future researchers.

At the conclusion of the baseline testing (or the initial evaluation session), the speech clinician makes several necessary decisions regarding the children who are accepted into a therapy program. Such matters as frequency of therapy, sound to be taught and mode of therapy (auditory or motor-oriented) are considered and decisions are made. In the context of a *behavioral evaluation,* decisions should also be made regarding the types of measures that will be employed to assess the child's behavior during therapy in order to determine the effectiveness of the selected therapy program. Several options are available to the clinician, but the different methods can be divided conveniently into intra-session and inter-session measures.

---

*Phonetic skills refer to the ability to produce the sound; phonemic skills refer to the integration of the available sounds in a linguistic system.

Intra-Session Measures

The level of performance of a child during a single therapy session can be compared to the behavior of a subject in a miniature learning theory study. In developing a therapy program, a clinician is hypothesizing that a given condition (e.g. *ear-training*) will have an effect upon the articulation profile of the child. Unfortunately, the effects of the program are rarely assessed during the course of treatment. The methodology of the experimental analysis of behavior (Brookshire, 1967; McReynolds, 1967) has not only contributed modification procedures to the clinical process but also produced a variety of measurement procedures and tools. Clinical speech pathology lends itself readily to the inclusion of these measurement devices.

Johnston and Harris (1968) have provided one system for categorizing and recording responses during the speech modification process:

(1) Records may be kept by the therapist during sessions.

(2) A tape recorder can be used to record all or part of the session, and the data transcribed later.

(3) An observer, trained in observation and recording methods, can record data on each session. (p. 45).

Utilizing a predetermined coding and scoring form, a speech clinician can obtain a record of the child's intra-session progress. These records, when transferred to a graph, provide an explicit, visual representation of the success of the program selected for the child. Mowrer (1969) has utilized logarithmic paper successfully in the recording of intra-session performance.

Stricker (1969) adopted a 40 response intra-session measure into her study of articulation therapy. The subjects were given therapy through a production mode following a sequence of isolation, syllable, word and phrase. During each session, a child received 40 test stimuli divided into 4 ten-item groups. As a standard procedure, the imitative mode of testing was used at all levels of therapy. A child was retained at a stage of therapy until he scored 32 correct responses out of the 40 items in one session. When he reached this criterion score, the next point in the therapy sequence was initiated. For example, a child who was working on a sound in the initial word position could not move to the medial or final word position until he obtained a score of 32 correct items on the intra-session measure.

Huston (1968) developed ten-item intra-session measures which consisted of four lists of words that contained the /s/ in the word initial position, the position selected for training in her study. Three of the ten-item lists were presented to the subjects during imitative training, and one list was reserved for the spontaneous phase of the therapy program. The approach used by Huston illustrated the application of intra-session measures developed according to the learning task presented to the child. The task for the children in this study was to learn the correct production of the /s/ in the initial position of nonsense words. Consequently, the test for generalization was designed to study the degree of *transfer* of correct productions from training stimuli to similar items.

The procedures and methods for recording intra-session changes (Mowrer, 1969; Johnston and Harris, 1968; Stricker, 1969; Huston, 1968) reflect the adaptability of such measures to the individual child and to the therapy program. Although equipment such as event recorders or digital counters can be easily incorporated into the process of taking such measures, simple plus and minus signs or tally marks can be equally effective for recording correct or incorrect behavior. The degree to which the intra-session measure assesses programs or generalization is a much more critical variable than the scoring procedure. Only an in-depth analysis of the articulatory behavior can accurately determine the form of measure; the scoring device or procedure should be determined by the availability of equipment to the clinician. The intra-session measures should be devised in such a way that they are a natural part of the therapy program and provide the clinician with a constant record of the articulatory status of the child through each level of the therapy program.

Inter-Session Measures

Inter-session measures refers to the degree to which a child has retained his level of production between sessions. Such measures are usually administered at the beginning of a session and not between two sessions as the name implies. Attempting to measure the skill maintained by a child from session-to-session can assist the clinician in determining the effectiveness of the therapy program and in making necessary adjustments in the program. This type of testing is extremely important for group therapy in which the children may be functioning at different levels of production. A child may even show a spurt of growth with a sound not being taught which may necessitate a change in the therapy program.

The sound production tasks (SPT) developed by Shelton and his associates (Elbert, *et al.*, 1967; Shelton *et al.*, 1967) are probably the best examples of inter-session measures. Originally designed as tools for research, they can serve as excellent models for a simple, quick method for obtaining a continuous record of a child's progress in therapy. The sound production tasks were developed according to McDonald's phonetic context theory (1964). There are thirty items in each SPT for each sound. The thirty items are randomly arranged three times to reduce a learning effect on the test scores. Sampling of different linguistic contexts is also included in the construction of the tasks. Each sound is sampled in isolation, in four nonsense syllables (two CV forms and two VC forms), thirteen-word and two-word constructs and twelve sentences. In the word and sentence constructs, the sound is tested in the environment of the most frequently occurring consonants. Thus, the phonetic contexts were selected with a rationale that relates to linguistic behavior. The SPT's are presented to the child through the imitative mode of presentation and scoring is on a right (+) and wrong (0) basis. Thus, the examiner can establish a criterion of completely accurate production and maintain the standard from session to session. Table II presents an example of one random arrangement for the phoneme /r/

The SPT approach to inter-session testing provides a rich variety of clinical information to the therapist in planning an articulation program for children. A clinician can vary the point during the session when the SPT is administered (Shelton *et al.*, 1967), the frequency with which it is given (i.e. daily or weekly) and can use it with groups as easily as with individual therapy (Freitag, Turton, Lea and Sautter, 1970). The SPT can be administered in approximately two minutes, allowing the therapist to obtain

TABLE II

EXAMPLE OF A SOUND PRODUCTION TASK FOR USE
AS AN INTER-SESSION MEASURE
RANDOM ARRANGEMENT II

/r/

1. Color the map red.
2. /ri/
3. /rae/
4. parking
5. The pig ran away.
6. Some rabbits are tame.
7. morethings
8. Bob read the book.
9. /ur/
10. darling
11. Did the bell ring?
12. Sit right here.
13. Does the dragon breathe red flames?
14. He can ride a bike.
15. party
16. parson
17. doorway
18. orbit
19. /r/
20. dearheart
21. firedog
22. fireman
23. He could write his name.
24. garnish
25. corrupt
26. Is the cake ready?
27. This ribbon is nice.
28. /ar/
29. He was running to school.
30. firezone

information on the sound being taught, as well as other sounds either within one or two sessions. The frequency with which the SPT is used is at the discretion of the clinician according to the needs of the children.

The particular form of inter-session measure, whether it be the SPT-type or some other innovative approach, should be selected, like the intra-session measures, to provide the therapist with sufficient information to make clinical judgements based upon data rather than upon subjective evaluations. Including inter-session measures in the evaluation process allows the clinician to decide whether to use them singly or with intra-session measures. For difficult cases, the clinician may decide to use the latter form of recording progress whereas the inter-session form may be more economical in terms of time for children who are showing rapid progress. These measures can also suggest to the therapist when to re-introduce some of the tests used in the original evaluation session.

SCORING AND ANALYZING ARTICULATION TESTS

Scoring Tests

The administration of an articulation test requires the selection of a scoring method which will yield maximum information for the effort. Articulation tests often have a built-in discrepancy between the scoring procedure and the method of interpreting the test results. A speech therapist will score the responses as omissions, substitutions and/or distortions and then attempt to describe the child's phonological skills by some numerical index. If we view the articulation test as the vehicle for determining the form of therapy, we should use an item-analysis approach in selecting the scoring procedure and the style of interpretation. Since we are dealing with phonological behavior, phonetic transcription is probably the most important scoring procedure that we can use during a pre-therapy evaluation session. Only phonetic transcription (either broad or narrow transcriptions as the child's behavior dictates) allows the tester to elicit sufficient information for an item analysis. Using phonetic transcription forces the therapist to reject the notion of a *distortion* and to realize that all productions of one sound for another are substitutions (Winitz, 1969).

The phonetic transcription makes possible a more detailed analysis of the relationship between the phonetic or linguistic context and the error. Phonetic laws (Heffner, 1950) clearly indicate that during correct productions, there is a systematic change in the production of the allophones of a phoneme as the context changes. Speech therapists should assume that the same holds true for misarticulations because the errors are probably controlled by the same phonological principles. A child who demonstrates a random pattern of error production by contexts within and among phonemes may have a more severe problem than the numerical score would indicate.

A decision regarding the scoring method for intra- and inter-session measures is generally dictated by the measure itself. Since these measures are designed for quick but frequent administration, they are best scored by simple procedures. For example, the sound production tasks are scored by a simple plus (+) or minus (−) system. The intra-session measures suggested by Johnston and Harris (1968) require only tally marks or other similar procedures. The use of phonetic transcription is not as critical with these measures because they are not incorporated into the process for placing a child into therapy or deciding with which sound to begin therapy. They do serve to verify the correctness of the decision but other procedures, particularly the frequency of administration, help to control for spurious or inaccurate results that may occur during one testing session.

Regardless of the scoring procedure selected, the speech therapist has a responsibility to maintain a high level of reliability. Although evidence exists (Siegel, 1962; Perrin, 1954; Stitt and Hunington, 1963) that the results for groups of clinicians are reliable, each clinician has a responsibility to determine his own degree of reliability and the phonemes that are the most difficult for him to score. Burger (1969) has demonstrated that therapists maintain their level of standards relative to each other and to themselves during the course of a therapy program. However, this was tested only for the sound production tasks which were not scored phonetically. A clinician cannot assume that he is a reliable tester. He must have evidence for the reliability, or the value of the articulation tests will diminish significantly.

Analyzing Articulation Tests

The next task for which the clinician is responsible is the analysis of the test results and the reduction of the scoring to a functional set of statements upon which therapy can be predicated. There are several procedures available to the clinician, all of which have inherent problems and should be used in conjunction with each other.

The simplest form of analysis is to reduce the responses to a numerical or percentile index that can be compared to a norm. This procedure is, however, only a screening procedure at best and yields virtually no information on the error pattern or the sounds that should receive therapy first. But this procedure can be of value in communicating with parents or with other professionals who can readily understand a quasi-mathematical statement of severity.

An analysis of phoneme errors based upon a substitution, distortion or omission scoring system yields slightly more information. When based upon a three-item test alone, this type of analysis can only be considered as tentative and of dubious value for determining the nature of the therapy program. Speech pathology has not produced evidence that a child with a predominance of substitutions in his pattern has a less severe problem than another child of the same age who usually omits the same sound. More importantly, we have not generated different therapy programs for each of these types of children. Consequently, without additional information, an ommission-substitution-distortion analysis is merely a more sophisticated form of the numerical index approach.

A popular method of analyzing articulation test results is to evaluate the child according to the norms of correct production for phonemes by age. Therapy is then structured according to the *easiest* sound for a child of a particular age to produce which is not yet in his repertoire. Not only does clinical experience suggest the weakness of this approach, but often it is done incorrectly. A complete comparison of a child to a norm should include a description of the sounds used correctly and the percentage of correctness for those sounds not yet acquired. An examination of the appendix of Templin's (1957) monograph clearly indicates that at any given age, children produce virtually all phonemes at a given level of success. A true age comparison should account for the percentage of correctness for defective phonemes when making norm comparisons.

The above-mentioned forms of analyses tend to ignore the error pattern which is the behavior that will be changed during the course of therapy. Speech clinicians frequently perform *ad hoc* error pattern analyses when they describe a child's problem as "predominantly plosive for fricative substitutions." Essentially, this form of analysis attempts to determine the broad phonological rules that control or characterize the child's articulatory error pattern. When performing this type of analysis, the clinician should be responding to three questions:

(1) Can the child produce the sound units of English regardless of the degree of correctness?

(2) Which phonemic features are present or absent in his articulation profile?

(3) Is there some basic phonological principle that appears to be controlling the misarticulations and which could be critical to the child's improvement?

The answer to the first question focuses on the ability of the child to produce the phonetic features of the language as they appear in sound units. At this level of analysis, the clinician is concerned only with the child's manipulation of the articulators to produce a sound that a listener perceives as being within the limits of English phonemes. Table III illustrates this part of the pattern analysis. The child (R.W.) whose pattern is depicted therein was a subject in a study by Park (1968). At the time of the study, he was a five-year-, two-month-old kindergartner with normal hearing, intelligence, medical and social history, with no previous experience in therapy. The analysis in Table III is based upon a broad phonetic scoring of R.W.'s responses to the 223-item test (Table I).

All of the basic consonant phonemes were produced by R.W. prior to therapy. Some of the sounds (e.g. the /r/) were produced correctly only in isolation; however, the /r/ phoneme errors were all *r-colored.* This child could be described as having adequate phonetic capabilities, i.e. he produces the fundamental articulatory movements of English regardless of whether the sound was used correctly as a phoneme or as a substitute for other sounds. Based upon this level of analysis, it would seem unlikely that a phonetic placement or drill approach would be necessary to teach him how to make sounds. The skill is already present.

Table IV presents the analysis of R.W.'s production according to phonemic accuracy or correctness. The sounds included in Table IV are those that the child produced correctly for each stimulus. As indicated in the table, this type of analysis reveals that the child does not produce labio-dental phonemes in terms of place of articulation. Both of these place categories exist only in conjunction with frication in English, and the child does not produce any fricative except for the glottal /h/. Consequently,

TABLE III

PRE-THERAPY *PHONETIC FEATURE* DISPLAY FOR SUBJECT R.W.
DISREGARDING CORRECTNESS

	Labial	Labio-dental	Lingua-dental	Lingua-alveolar	Lingua-palatal	Lingua-velar	Glottal
Nasal	m			n		ŋ	
Plosive	p–b			t–d		k–g	
Fricative		f–v	θ–ǯ	s–z	ʃ–ʒ		h
Affricate					t͡ʃ–d͡ʒ		
Lateral				l			
Semi-vowel	w				r–j		

Analysis: All features of English in phonetic combinations

phonemic errors along the parameter of frication should probably be considered to be the critical variable in this child's pattern rather than place features. Of particular interest is the correct production of the affricates. Depending upon results of auditory discrimination testing,* the restriction of the error pattern to fricatives and glides suggests an auditory orientation to therapy.

Examination of Table V † provides more information on the

*Since this child was part of a research project, only the 223-item test and the sound production tasks were administered pre-therapy. Auditory discrimination and deep-testing were not performed. This analysis of R.W. was not performed pre-therapy. His change during therapy led to the development of this type of analysis.

†For the sake of ease of presentation, the liquids were eliminated from Table V.

TABLE IV

PHONEMES PRODUCED CORRECTLY BY SUBJECT R. W.
PRE-THERAPY

	Labial	Labio-dental	Lingua-dental	Lingua-alveolar	Lingua-palatal	Lingua-velar	Glottal
Nasal	m			n		ŋ	
Plosive	p—b			t—d		k—g	h
Fricative							
Affricate					tʃ—dʒ		
Lateral							
Semi-vowel	w				j		

Analysis: Place features of the labio-dental and the lingua-dental not produced.
Manner features of fricative (except /h/) and lateralization not produced.

fricatives which allows the clinician to synthesize the error pattern with greater precision. R.W.'s *phonological-error rule* could be stated as the substitution of a stop or affricate for a fricative. Although there are obvious exceptions to this rule, it permeates the fricative system of this child. Thus, the clinician can show additional support for an auditory approach to therapy because an hypothesis could be developed that the child does not discriminate between fricatives and affricates. That is, the phonological cue of frication evokes a stop plus frication or stop response on the part of the child.

The sound selection process becomes a somewhat different

TABLE V

ANALYSIS OF ERROR RESPONSES OF SUBJECT R. W.
ON THE 223–ITEM TEST

	ʃ	θ	v	s	ʒ	z	f	ð̸
Spontaneous Words	tʃ	f	b	—	*	d		*
	tʃ	—	b			d	—	d
	tʃ	tʃ	b	ts			ts	*
Imitated Words	tʃ	s	b	—	*	d		v
	tʃ	ts	d	X	dʒ	dʒ	s	dʒ
	tʃ	ts	dʒ	ts	dʒ	dʒ	ts	z
Isolation					z			v
Imitated Phrases	tʃ	h	b	—	*	X		
	tʃ	—	d	ts	dʒ	X	—	dʒ
	tʃ	ts	dʒ	ts	dʒ	X	t	dʒ

* No stimulus is available for these items

General "Error Rule": Substitute stop or affricate for fricative.

problem when the articulation deviances are reduced to an error-rule. The clinician should make the decision according to which sound(s) will effect the most generalization of correct productions from one phoneme to another. Stated differently, sound selection should be based upon a prediction as to which sound changes will most disrupt the prevailing error rule. The / θ / was the target sound for R.W. because it was the phoneme selected for study by Park (1968). However, the choice can be justified because it combines the place feature of dentalization with frication, providing economy of therapy.

In the case of R.W., phoneme class generalization produced improvement of the / ʃ /, as well as other fricatives. A significant clinical sign of the disruption of the error rule was the overgeneralization to the /tʃ / phoneme. Prior to the study, R.W. produced the /tʃ / correctly at a 100 percent rate. As the error rule was modified and, specifically, as he eliminated the /tʃ / for / ʃ / substitution, he reversed the substitution pattern. The overgeneralization resulted in an / ʃ / for /tʃ / substitution pattern.

The determination of the linguistic context as the base-point for therapy can also be made from this type of analysis. Examination of data, as found in Table V plus an item analysis of sound production tasks administered pre-therapy, can provide the clinician with information regarding the child's skills in nonsense syllables, isolated productions, words and phrases. A clinician can find the linguistic context that appears to facilitate correct productions of the phoneme. Again, drawing a parallel with phonetic context theories, the therapist should assume that the consistency of misarticulation may also be a function of the grammatical form in which the sound occurs.

This relationship between sound and linguistic context was exemplified by another subject in the Park (1968) study who showed little change during the course of therapy despite a higher level of correct production than the other subjects for the / θ /. Analysis of the sound production tasks administered pre-therapy indicated that she was already producing the target phoneme at the word and the phrase levels of linguistic context at the beginning of the therapy program. Consequently, the first few months of therapy merely reinforced her existing behavior rather than upgrading her phonological skills. The phrase section of the 223-item test (Table I) did not provide a sufficient number of stimuli to indicate to the clinician that therapy should begin at the higher levels of linguistic context.

The error pattern analysis, in conjunction with the normative and numerical index analysis, can provide the clinician with a relatively total system for synthesizing the articulation skills of a child. Although the total analysis appears to be time-consuming, the time potentially saved during therapy justifies the effort. Furthermore, the work can be performed in the absence of the child, reducing the need for additional clinician-child interactions during the decision making process. The analysis task proposed herein follows the spirit of the following statement by Van Riper and Irwin (1958):

> When the articulation case presents himself to us for therapy we must do more than try to determine the causal factors that initiated the problem or contributed to its severity. We must also scrutinize his speech to determine the nature of the deviant behavior. We must discover the articulatory errors that make his speech unacceptable. Our therapeutic task will be to eliminate them and replace them with the standard sounds of our language. Unless we do this analyzing, we will work blindly and so will the case. (p.48).

THE PROCESS OF GENERALIZATION*

Possible Forms of Generalization

Speech clinicians have long recognized that generalization is often a natural consequence of the modification process. It is not uncommon for a clinician to remediate one member of a cognate pair (e.g. the /s/) and not the other because the generalization effect of therapy will tend to improve the other member (/z/) without specific procedures (Elbert, Shelton and Ardnt, 1967). Another approach is to introduce the second sound before the first sound has reached criterion in order to hasten the process of generalization. Generalization during articulation therapy, however, may involve several other possible forms.

Research has demonstrated that generalization can occur across training procedures (McLean, 1970) and across word positions (Powell and McReynolds, 1967). Park (1968) and Stricker (1969) have shown that phonetically similar sounds, other than cognates, improve during the course of therapy. Freitag, Turton, Lea and

---

*Generalization as described in this section refers to the increase in the number of correct productions of a phoneme either in a context in which it has not received therapy or as a result of therapy with a different phoneme.

Sautter (1970) reported that during the period of 22 weeks of therapy, two children showed improvement with phonetically dissimilar sounds. Although this finding may be spurious or reflect an experimenter bias, it points to the possibility of a more pervasive form of generalization. Placing a child into articulation therapy for one sound may actually affect his total articulation profile. The clinician perhaps presents two *messages* to the child: (1) the environment will no longer accept his misarticulations and (2) the skills that he is acquiring to change one sound can be applied to other misarticulated phonemes. Especially in the imitative phases of therapy, the child may be concentrating on the experimenter's articulation in a way that he has never concentrated before. He is likely to become aware of sounds other than the target sound and to become aware of articulatory differences which he has never noticed before. Essentially, a clinician should be able to expect generalization according to phonetic variables, linguistic variables and learning variables.

Sound Selection and Generalization

At the completion of the analysis of the articulation testing, a clinician should have sufficient information to allow not only for the selection of the first sound to be given therapy but also the order in which all sounds will receive therapy. Sound selection could be viewed as the point in the development of a therapy program when phonetic features are used to determine the sound sequence for therapy. In the case of R. W. (Tables III–V), the analysis indicated that the phonetic class of fricatives was defective and that affricates or plosives were usually substituted for the fricatives. When ordering the sounds for therapy, a clinician could then look at the articulation test with the following objectives in mind: (1) to facilitate increased correct production of fricative phonemes with a minimum amount of therapy and (2) to modify the *error rule* apparently governing the misarticulations. From a learning point of view, the fricatives could be described as a response class with expected phonetic similarities and inherent defective features. Therapy for one sound should then be expected to affect the entire class.

Evaluating R. W.'s defective fricatives by phonetic variables, assuming the /θ/ as the initial sound for therapy, could be performed according to the following logic. /θ/ is a voiceless, lingua-dental, broad fricative. It is highly visual and can be taught easily in a restricted number of words. In R. W.'s profile it was not used consistently as a substitute for another sound. Comparing it to the other defective fricatives, generalization can be expected to /ð/ as its cognate. Improvement in /f/ and /v/ should occur because they share the features of dentalization and broad frication. /ʃ/ and /ʒ/ share with /θ/ the features of frontal lingual placement and broad frication. /s/ and /z/, the narrow fricatives, share features of lingual movement and frication with the /θ/ and do not have a highly consistent substitution.

A possible sequence of sounds for therapy for the fricative could then be as follows: /θ/ and /ð/, /f/, /v/, /s/, /z/, /ʃ/ and /ʒ/. Continuous evaluation of the child's progress through intra- and inter-session measures would confirm the sequence selected as well as suggesting modifications. Stricker (1969) noted in her study that for some children, other sounds improved faster than the target sound during the course of therapy. She suggested that perhaps the other sounds should either be incorporated into the therapy program or should replace the target sound as the phoneme receiving emphasis.

The suggested rank order should not be considered as a fixed sequence but only as illustrative of the principle that potential phoneme generalization should be considered in the development of a therapy program. The selection of a sound should never be determined out of the context of the other defective sounds. Disregarding the other sounds is a clinical rejection of the phonological rules of the language and phonemic development.*

Other Forms of Generalization

Generalization facilitated by learning conditions and by linguistic contexts are not within the scope of this chapter. However, the recent literature in these subjects should be taken into account

---

*See Crocker (1969) as an example of one potential sequence of the development of phonological rules.

by the speech clinician. McLean (1970) has evaluated procedures for developing generalization by controlling the learning conditions. Winitz (1969) has presented a set of procedures for developing a programmed approach to articulation therapy. Awareness of these procedures should help the clinician to develop a therapy program for children according to their articulation profiles and not by predetermined approaches such as *ear training* or *sensorimotor training.*

SUMMARY

This chapter was concerned with a concept of articulation testing extending beyond the traditional diagnostic functions of the therapy program. Articulation testing was viewed as a function of the behavioral evaluation of the phonological system of a child. The evaluation procedures should be maintained throughout therapy as intra- and inter-session measures. A clinician has a responsibility to analyze test results in order to program therapy according to the child's needs. Generalization should be viewed as an integral part of the program predicated upon the child's defective sounds and the phonological rules affecting the misarticulations. Sound selection should be a process of selecting the sequence in which the sounds are taught and not selection of each sound in isolation from other sounds.

REFERENCES

Brookshire, R. H.: Speech pathology and the experimental analysis of behavior. J Speech Hear Disord, 32:215-227, 1967.

Burger, M. S.: Temporal stability of reliability judgements of articulation. Unpublished Master's thesis, Bowling Green State University, 1969.

Carter, E. T., and Buck, M.: Prognostic testing for functional articulation disorders among children in the first grade. J Speech Hear Disord, 23:124-133, 1958.

Crocker, J. R.: A phonological model of children's articulation competence. J Speech Hear Disord, 34:203-213, 1969.

Darley, F. L.: Diagnosis and Appraisal of Communication Disorders. Englewood Cliffs, Prentice-Hall, Inc., 1964.

Elbert, M., Shelton, R. L., and Ardnt, W. B.: A task for evaluation of articulation change: I. Development of methodology. J Speech Hear Res, 10:281-289, 1967.

Farquahar, M.: Prognostic value of imitative and auditory discrimination test. J Speech Hear Disord, 26:342-347, 1961.

Freitag, W., Turton, L. J., Lea, J. P., and Sautter, C. Z.: Effects of Scheduling upon Articulation Therapy: Phase 1. Research report, Ohio Department of Education, 1970.

Goldman, R., and Fristoe, M.: Goldman – Fristoe Test of Articulation. Circle Pines, American Guidance Service, Inc., 1969.

Heffner, R. M. S.: General Phonetics. Madison, University of Wisconsin Press, 1950.

Huston, J. K.: The evaluation of a procedure of model phonemic contrast training. Unpublished Master's thesis, University of Kansas, 1968.

Johnson, W., Darley, F. L., and Spriestersbach, D. C.: Diagnostic Methods in Speech Pathology. New York, Harper & Row, 1963.

Johnston, M., and Harris, F. R.: Observation and recording of verbal behavior in remedial speech work. In H. N. Sloane, Jr. and B. D. Macaulay (Eds.): Operant Procedures in Remedial Speech and Language Training. Boston, Houghton Mifflin, 1968.

McDonald, E. T.: Articulation Testing and Treatment: A Sensory – Motor Approach. Pittsburgh, Stanwix House, Inc., 1964.

McLean, J.: Extending stimulus control of phoneme articulation by operant techniques. In F. L. Girardeau and J. E. Spradlin (Eds.): A Functional Approach to Speech and Language. ASHA Monographs Number 14, 1970.

McReynolds, L. V.: Verbal sequence discrimination training for language impaired children. J Speech Hear Disord, 32:249-256, 1967.

Mowrer, D. E.: Evaluating speech therapy through precision recording. J Speech Hear Disord, 34:239-244, 1969.

Park, K. S.: The effects of speech therapy upon the articulation profiles of kindergarten children. Unpublished Master's thesis, University of Kansas, 1968.

Perrin, E.: Rating of defective speech by trained and untrained observers. J Speech Hear Disord, 19:48-51, 1954.

Powell, J., and McReynolds, L. V.: A procedure for testing position generalization from articulation training. J Speech Hear Res, 12:629-645, 1969.

Shelton, R. L., Elbert, M., and Ardnt, W. B.: A task for evaluation of articulation change: II. Comparison of task scores during baseline and lesson series testing. J Speech Hear Res, 10:578-586, 1967.

Siegel, G. M.: Experienced and inexperienced articulation examiners. J Speech Hear Disord, 27:28-35, 1962.

Sommers, R. K., Leiss, R. H., Delp, M. A., Gerber, A., Fundrella, D., Smith, R. M., Revucky, M. V., Ellis, D. and Haley, V. A.: Factors related to the effectiveness of articulation therapy for kindergarten, first and second grade children. J Speech Hear Res, 10:428-437, 1967.

Stricker, F. M.: The effects of therapy based upon phonetic context on phonetically similar sounds. Unpublished Master's thesis, Bowling Green

State University, 1969.

Stitt, C. L., and Hunington, D.: Reliability of judgments of articulation proficiency. J Speech Hear Res, 6:49-56, 1963.

Templin, M. C.: Certain Language Skills in Children. Minneapolis, University of Minnesota Press, 1957.

Van Riper, C., and Irwin, J. V.: Voice and Articulation. Englewood Cliffs, Prentice-Hall, Inc., 1958.

Winitz, H.: Articulatory Acquisition and Behavior. New York, Appleton-Century-Crofts, Inc., 1969.

CHAPTER X

EVALUATING ARTICULATION THERAPY

LESTER F. AUNGST and EUGENE T. McDONALD

It is well known that disorders of articulation comprise the majority of all speech disorders and an even larger proportion of the caseloads of the majority of speech clinicians who work in public school settings. Less well publicized, but equally well known among speech clinicians, is that, while many persons with defective articulation improve rapidly with articulation therapy, there are others whose speech remains defective even after years of therapy. It also has been speculated that some persons, especially younger children, who respond quickly to therapy might develop normal articulation even without therapy. Furthermore, practicing speech clinicians often have expressed dissatisfaction with currently used methods of articulation therapy.

In view of the foregoing, it is remarkable to find that experimental studies designed to evaluate various therapeutic techniques and procedures for treating disorders of articulation have been rare. The majority of studies involving evaluation of therapy have been concerned primarily with different ways of *scheduling* the treatment. Related to problems of scheduling are those studies which have investigated whether treatment produced significantly greater improvement than no treatment. In this chapter we shall review a selection of these studies, as well as those few studies which have been directed toward comparisons between therapeutic techniques and approaches. We shall conclude with a discussion of some critical issues involved in evaluating the

NOTE: Portions of this chapter were prepared under a grant from the U. S. Office of Education.

effectiveness of articulation therapy.

A number of the studies reviewed below have dealt with speech improvement methods rather than speech therapy methods. Although the rationale for a particular method of instruction might apply equally to speech improvement and to speech therapy, the differences lie in the persons toward whom the instruction is directed and in the sometimes subtle distinction between instructional, as contrasted with therapeutic, and clinical interaction. In most cases, speech improvement instruction is given indiscriminately to an entire classroom of children or to a large group of persons with minor speech deviations, while speech therapy involves more intensified and individualized interaction only with those who seem to need this special help. Studies dealing with the evaluation of speech improvement methods are of interest here, but the results are not necessarily applicable to speech therapy with more selective populations.

THERAPY VERSUS NO THERAPY

Employment of a control group which receives no treatment is a standard experimental technique to account for behavioral changes which might be attributed to factors in the experimental procedure other than the particular treatments being studied. Another important use of control groups arises in studies of the articulatory proficiency of children in whom normal maturation may not be complete. Thus there are two types of questions which may be answered by studies of therapy versus no therapy. One concerns whether therapy is better than nothing, while the other involves the advisability of some form of intervention in developmental processes.

Wilson (1954) evaluated a speech improvement program for kindergarten children. Classrooms were selected at random, with 128 children receiving speech improvement instruction from their classroom teacher for 12 weeks and 114 children receiving no speech instruction. Pre-test and post-test scores were obtained by means of a three-position test of articulation designed especially for the study. Wilson found that reduction in the mean number of articulation errors was related to the experimental treatment (instruction) and that articulation errors were reduced for sounds not included in the lessons.

Butler (1960) assigned 353 kindergarten children to nine experimental (speech improvement instruction) and five control (no instruction) groups. Comparisons of pre-test and post-test articulation results showed the experimental groups averaged 47 per cent corrected, while the control groups averaged 25 per cent corrected.

Holbrook (1954) divided 42 university students of Oriental descent into two groups. The experimental group received training by means of tape-recorded speech exercises, while the control group was not trained. Pre-training and post-training recordings of the subjects' speech were evaluated for sound substitutions. The experimental group showed significant improvement in terms of the mean number of sound substitutions.

The effect of creative activities on the articulation of 32 children with speech disorders was studied by McIntyre (1958). The children were divided into two closely matched groups of equal number. The experimental group participated in the program of creative activities with 185 other children, while the control group did not. Pre-experiment and post-experiment articulation scores were obtained with a special articulation test which had been constructed by McWilliams (1953) to test speech sounds according to their relative frequency in the English language. Significant improvement was shown for more children in the experimental group than in the control group.

The consistent finding of these studies that some form of treatment is superior to no treatment is supported by other studies which have included a no-treatment condition as part of their experimental designs (e.g. Barnett, 1948; Chisum, 1969; Pfeifer, 1958; Sommers, 1961, 1962a, 1970; Ventura, Ingebo and Wolmut, 1960). These findings, however, do not account for the clinical fact that some persons do not seem to benefit from the treatment they receive, while other individuals improve without treatment, nor do they account for the fact that some persons make greater improvement than others under the same treatment conditions. Studies which have attempted solutions to the problem of differential responses to treatment usually have been focused upon the predictive value of certain conditions such as intelligence or socio-economic status or of certain tests such as those of Carter and Buck (1958) and Van Riper and Erickson (1969). Prognostic studies usually have been directed toward questions of case selection rather than case management. Effectiveness of therapy, when it has been considered as a variable in predictive studies, has been employed as a criterion for evaluating the prognostic indicators under study (e.g. Sommers *et al* ., 1967).

SCHEDULING

Studies of scheduling usually involve questions concerning the frequency or duration of therapy. We also have included here studies dealing with group versus individual therapy because this question has been included in some of the scheduling studies, and for some professional workers it seems to be viewed primarily as a problem of scheduling.

Sommers and his co-workers have conducted a series of studies involving questions of scheduling, among others. In the first of these studies (Sommers *et al.,* 1961), a population of first grade children was randomly sampled to receive (a) speech improvement, (b) speech therapy for nine months or (c) speech therapy for three months. In addition to these three groups, 25 children with severe disorders of articulation received both speech improvement and speech therapy for nine months. Children who were not selected to receive training served as controls. A three-position test of articulation for ten sounds was used to measure speech gains. Subjects who received nine months of speech therapy made significantly greater gains than either their controls or the speech improvement group. Subjects who received nine months of speech improvement made significantly greater gains than their control groups and did as well (no significant difference) as the group who received only three months of speech therapy. Subjects who received only three months of speech therapy did not differ in speech gains from their controls. Combined speech therapy and speech improvement for nine months produced significantly greater gains than nine months of speech improvement alone.

In a follow-up study of a second group of first grade children,

Sommers *et al.* (1962a) found that speech improvement was better than no instruction and that nine months of speech improvement was better than 16 weeks of speech improvement in the middle of the school term. Continuing speech improvement training into the second grade with children who had received training in first grade resulted in no significant improvement in articulation when these children were compared with second graders who had received training in first grade only.

In a study of group versus individual therapy, Sommers *et al.* (1966) randomly selected 240 second, fourth and sixth grade children, all of whom had average or better intelligence quotients, functional articulation problems and normal hearing. The children were grouped according to grade level and defectiveness of articulation. Half of the children in each group received individual therapy and half received group therapy. Pre-therapy and post-therapy testing was done using McDonald's Deep Test of Articulation. At the end of the eight month experimental period, it was found that group therapy was as effective as individual therapy for all subjects regardless of grade level and severity of the articulation problem.

In a study of the efficacy of articulation therapy with retarded children, Sommers *et al* (1970) selected 180 educable mentally retarded subjects on the basis of *good* versus *poor* prognostic scores on the Carter/Buck Test and on the basis of moderate versus severe degrees of articulatory defectiveness based upon a version of McDonald's Picture Deep Test of Articulation (McDonald, 1964). The 45 subjects in each of the four resulting categories were then randomly assigned to three experimental conditions: (a) group articulation therapy scheduled one time per week, (b) group articulation therapy scheduled four times per week and (c) control (no therapy). Comparison of pre-therapy and post-therapy Deep Test results indicated that both experimental groups showed improvement while the control group did not; however, only the improvements made by those subjects receiving therapy four times per week were significantly different from the control group scores. It is interesting to note that, contrary to the findings of an earlier study (Sommers *et al.*, 1967) conducted with children of normal intelligence, neither prognostic scores nor severity of misarticulation were related to the improvement made by these mentally retarded subjects.

Also studying educable mentally retarded children, Pfeifer (1958) found that subjects who received speech therapy improved significantly compared to subjects who received no therapy; however, no significant differences were found between the effects of group therapy and the effects of individual therapy.

Weaver and Wollersheim (1964) found a block system of scheduling to be superior to an intermittent scheduling of speech cases.

COMPARISON OF THERAPY
APPROACHES OR TECHNIQUES

Although the studies discussed above provide valuable information for speech clinicians, it also is important to study variables occurring within therapy sessions. Such studies include those which attempt to evaluate particular therapeutic procedures or which compare one or more therapeutic techniques or approaches. For example, a number of the studies previously cited involved speech improvement; it is logical that the effectiveness of speech improvement and speech therapy should be compared. One such study was reviewed in the previous section (Sommers *et al.*, 1961).

Barnett (1958) compared three methods of teaching voice and diction to college freshmen. Seventy subjects were divided into three experimental groups to be taught by ear training, phonetic or oral reading approaches. A control group of 20 subjects received no training. Judges' ratings of gross speaking performance and the articulation of specific sounds found no differences among the three experimental groups, but a significant difference was found between the experimental subjects and the control subjects.

Reiner (1959) compared a phonetic method and an imitative method of teaching speech sounds to college students with functional disorders of articulation. Pre-training and post-training tape-recordings were evaluated by a panel of three speech teachers using a seven-point rating scale. Imitative training was found to be more effective than phonetic training.

Holland and Matthews (1963) investigated the application of

teaching machine concepts to speech training. Three different programs were prepared for using a teaching machine procedure of teaching discrimination of /s/. Twenty-seven children who misarticulated /s/ were divided into three groups matched for their ability to discriminate /s/. One group of nine subjects was assigned to each of the teaching programs. One of the programs proved to be definitely superior to the others in improving sound discrimination, but no significant differences in post-training articulation ability was found among the three groups.

Webb and Siegenthaler (1957) used six different aural stimulation methods to teach six new sounds to normal speaking children. A subject's score was the number of correct productions among the several sounds and among the six methods. Verbal instruction plus evaluation by a judge proved to be the best method of instruction.

Lieblich (1964) conducted a similar study in which three French sounds were taught to 108 elementary school children using three methods: phonetic placement, stimulation and a multiple method. Initial training, relearning and recall were measured. No method was found to be superior for teaching all three sounds, but "certain methods showed definite superiority for individual sounds."

Gerber (1966) compared the achievement of carry-over for the /r/ sound with two treatment procedures. Sixteen subjects who scored at least 60 per cent correct on a short version of the McDonald Deep Test of Articulation, and who scored no better than 60 per cent correct production of /r/ in a sample of spontaneous speech, were divided into an experimental and a control group which were matched for age and scoring on the spontaneous speech test. The experimental group engaged in individual, self-administered therapy involving simultaneous self-evaluation using the Echorder for 20 minutes twice a week for nine weeks. The control group received traditional articulation therapy in groups of three to five children twice weekly in sessions lasting 30 minutes. Comparison of the mean percentage of correct production of /r/ on a post-treatment, spontaneous speech test indicated that the experimental subjects made significantly greater improvement than the control subjects. Also, four of the eight experimental subjects achieved a previously determined criterion for carry-over, while no control subjects achieved this criterion.

McDonald and Aungst (1967) conducted a three year field study to compare the improvement made in speech sound production by children from grades three, four, five and six under three conditions: *sensory-motor* therapy, *traditional* articulation therapy and no therapy. Twenty-nine public school speech clinicians and 843 children with disorders of articulation participated in various phases of the study. Results were reported only for those subjects who misarticulated /s/ or /r/. Neither the traditional nor the sensory-motor approach to therapy was found to be clearly superior for obtaining improvement in articulation during therapy. It was found, however, that regression in articulation scores occurred over a summer of no therapy following a year of traditional therapy, whereas comparable regression did not occur following a year of sensory-motor therapy. The results of the study also suggested that (1) two distinct phases of articulatory development may exist, a *programming* phase and a *practicing* phase, (2) a deep test of articulation may reflect the degree to which a child is programmed for the correct production of a sound, (3) after a certain level of programming and practice is reached, a child may make comparable progress with or without therapy and (4) improvement in speech sound production appears to be associated with an interaction of pre-therapy levels of programming, specific error sound, therapy method and clinician.

The results of these studies suggest that the method or approach employed in a treatment program influences the outcomes of that program; however, the findings are not as clear nor as convincing as we might wish.

DISCUSSION

Most research on articulation is open to considerable criticism, in terms of both its conceptualization and its execution (Sommers, 1967; Locke, 1968). We would like to call attention to some of these criticisms, adding a few concerns of our own, relevant to evaluations of articulation therapy. We do not mean to imply by any exclusions that other criticisms and concerns are less valid than those we mention.

A central problem in evaluating articulation therapy is the selection of an appropriate criterion measure. There seem to be almost as many tests of articulation as there are studies. Traditional initial-medial-final-plus-blends tests yielding total scores and ignoring differences among the various speech sounds are of questionable value, particularly in evaluating therapy which often is directed toward a single phoneme. The development of *deep tests* of articulation (McDonald, 1959, 1964a, 1964b, 1968) has proved valuable for research, as well as diagnosis and treatment, by providing a measure of the variability in the articulation of each phoneme across a representative sample of phonetic contexts. Assessing the articulation of each phoneme separately is important because one phoneme is not the same as another and there is reason to believe that the learning of one phoneme may differ in many ways from the learning of another phoneme.

Even more important than the particular test employed is the tester who employs it; for example, no competent audiologist would measure hearing with an uncalibrated or unreliable audiometer. In assessing articulation, it is the ear of the examiner which is the measuring instrument, yet few studies have reported the reliability of the examiner's judgements or how that reliability was obtained, not to mention the validity of the judgments. Furthermore, it is disappointing to find that the *norm* for interjudge agreement would appear to be less than 85 per cent (Irwin and Krafchick, 1965).

Perhaps the most overlooked variable in studying the effectiveness of articulation therapy is the clinician. It is curious that there seems to be more interest in the role of the parent as a significant therapeutic variable (e.g. Lillywhite, 1948; McWilliams, 1959; Sommers *et al.*, 1959, 1962b; Tufts, 1959; Wood, 1946, 1948) than in the role of the clinician. While there has been little research on the topic, the speech pathology literature contains many suggestions that the clinician constitutes an important variable in the therapeutic situation. In our own research (McDonald and Aungst, 1967), we found evidence suggesting considerable variability in effectiveness within and among speech clinicians. Some clinicians obtained better results in teaching one sound than in teaching another; in teaching a given sound, some clinicians obtained better results with one therapy method, while another method seemed more effective for others; some clinicians obtained better results than others regardless of sound or method. Not only should clinician variability be taken into consideration when designing therapy evaluation studies, but the basis for the variability also should be investigated. Is it related to the personality of the clinician, the clinician's training, the pairing of a particular clinician with a particular client, some as yet unsuspected factors or some combination of these?

The *subject* also constitutes an important variable when evaluating the effectiveness of therapy. If subjects who receive treatment are drawn from the same population as subjects who improve without treatment, then the effectiveness of the treatment cannot be clearly determined. Subjects who improve without treatment are essentially normal. What is needed is a means of assuring that subjects identified as defective have been drawn from a truly defective population. Because of the high proportion of false positive and false negative results, existing predictive measures such as the Carter-Buck test have limited value for general case-selection (Winitz, 1969) and are unsatisfactory for precise identification of research populations. More precise identification of the articulatory defective population should include identification of sub-groups within that population. Clinical observation suggests that a particular therapy approach may be more effective with one sub-group than another. If this is so, the identification of such sub-groups would be crucial for evaluating the effectiveness of therapy. All too often we find that attention to the results for a group of subjects taken as a whole has obscured quite different results for a sizable portion of the group. Responses to treatment which are at variance with those of the majority must be accounted for if we are to have a satisfactory evaluation of the effectiveness of that treatment.

The typical design of most of the studies we have reviewed involves an assessment of articulation at only two points in the study — before and again after a period of therapy. Rarely have there been attempts to evaluate the longer-term effects of therapy, namely *carry-over,* particularly following termination of therapy. Yet clinicians assert that attaining carry-over is perhaps the most difficult aspect of the therapeutic process and is the ultimate test of the effectiveness of therapy. It has been found that differences between the outcomes of different therapy approaches might not be revealed until the stability of therapy gains are determined following a period of no therapy (McDonald and Aungst, 1967).

In addition to assessing carry-over, it appears increasingly important to assess changes occurring during therapy. This is particularly so, if, as we strongly suspect, certain approaches or precedures are more effective during certain stages of therapy than during others. It is quite possible that, when learning to articulate a sound, a child must first be *programmed* for the distinctive features of that sound and then have *practice* in producing the sound and comparing his production with the programmed model. Therapy approaches appropriate for programming may not be appropriate for practice, and vice versa. Once a child reaches a certain level of programming and practice, he may continue to improve without further therapy. Furthermore, the several levels and the specific therapy procedures appropriate for each may vary depending upon the error sound. The research of Brungard (1961), among others, suggests that the several stages of learning a sound may be identified by performance on a deep test of articulation. These hypotheses, however, must be tested through further research.

While we do not consider this an exhaustive discussion of valid criticisms and concerns about evaluations of articulation therapy, none of the studies which we have cited has attended adequately to the problems we have mentioned. It is apparent that a concerted, continuing research effort is needed to better understand the nature of articulation, the nature of defective articulation and the nature of the therapeutic process, including the participants in that process.

We do not mean to suggest, however, that efforts to evaluate therapy should be suspended until some or all of the related problems have been solved. Rather, solving these problems may be hastened by appropriately taking them into account in studies of therapy, as suggested by Sommers (1967). Neither do we mean to suggest that the clinical practitioner cannot make a significant contribution to this area of study. Careful documentation of therapy can yield much useful information toward the solution of the problems that concern us. For example, the clinician who makes periodic, systematic assessments during therapy, using deep tests or measures such as those suggested by Shelton and his co-workers (Elbert *et al.,* 1967; Shelton *et al.,* 1967; Wright *et al.,* 1969) or by Mowrer (1969), not only obtains valuable information about the progress of his clients and about his own effectiveness, but also has information which should be valuable for a better understanding of the therapeutic process. Such information also might prove useful for evaluation of the measures themselves. Furthermore, if many cases of defective articulation are the result of arrested development (McDonald, 1964a), then information about learning which occurs during therapy may prove useful for a better understanding of learning which takes place during normal development. We *do* mean to suggest that cooperative research and continuing dialogue between researchers and clinicians can be mutually beneficial and well worth the effort; it seems to us the best way to improve both the quantity and the quality of evaluations of articulation therapy and ultimately to increase the effectiveness of articulation therapy for all those who need it.

REFERENCES

Barnett, W.: An experimental study in the teaching of voice and diction through ear training, phonetic and oral reading approaches. Speech Monogr, 15:142-154, 1948.

Brungard, M. O.: Effect of consistency of articulation of [r] and [s] on gains made with and without therapy. Ed.D. dissertation, Pennsylvania State University, 1961.

Butler, K.: An empirical investigation of speech improvement in the elementary school. ASHA, 2:372, 1960.

Carter, E., and Buck, M.: Prognostic testing for functional articulation disorders among children in the first grade. J Speech Hear Disord, 23:124-133, 1958.

Chisum, L., *et al.*: Relationship between remedial speech instruction activities and articulation change. Cleft Palate J., 6:57-64, 1969.

Elbert, M., *et al.:* A task for the evaluation of articulation change: I. Development of methodology. J Speech Hear Res, 10:281-288, 1967.

Gerber, A.: The achievement of /r/ carry-over through intensification of simultaneous auditory feedback. Pennsylvania Speech Hearing Assoc. Newsletter, 7, February, 1966.

Holbrook, A.: A study of the effectiveness of recorded articulation exercises. J Speech Hear Disord, 19:14-16, 1954.

Holland, A., and Matthews, J.: Application of teaching machine concepts to speech pathology and audiology. ASHA, 5:474-482, 1963.

Irwin, R. B., and Krafchick, I. P.: An audio-visual test for evaluating the ability to recognize phonetic errors. J Speech Hear Res, 8:281-290, 1965.

Lieblich, M.: Comparative effectiveness of methods of teaching correct production of sounds. ASHA, 6:395, 1964.

Lillywhite, H.: Make mother a clinician. J Speech Hear Disord, 13:61-66, 1948.

Locke, J. L.: Questionable assumptions underlying articulation research. J Speech Hear Disord, 33:112-116, 1968.

McDonald, E. T.: Rationale for a "deep test" of articulation. ASHA, 1:103, 1959.

McDonald, E. T.: Articulation Testing and Treatment: A Sensory-Motor Approach. Pittsburgh, Stanwix House, 1964a.

McDonald, E. T.: A Deep Test of Articulation. Pittsburgh, Stanwix House, 1964b.

McDonald, E. T.: A Screening Deep Test of Articulation. Pittsburgh, Stanwix House, 1968.

McDonald, E. T. and Aungst, L. F.: Evaluation of sensory-motor articulation therapy. Project Report, Research Grant No. C–55. Washington, Children's Bureau, DHEW, 1967.

McIntyre, B. M.: The effect of creative activities on the articulation skills of children with speech disorders. Speech Monogr, 25:42-48, 1958.

McWilliams, B. J.: An Experimental study of some of the components of intelligibility of the speech of adult cleft-palate patients. Ph.D. dissertation, University of Pittsburgh, 1953.

McWilliams, B. J.: Adult education program for mothers of children with speech handicaps. J Speech Hear Disord, 24:408-410, 1959.

Mowrer, D. E.: Evaluating speech therapy through precision recording. J Speech Hear Disord, 34:239-244, 1969.

Pfiefer, R. C.: An experimental analysis of individual and group speech therapy with educable institutionalized mentally retarded children. Ed.D. dissertation, Boston University, 1958.

Reiner, K. S.: A comparison of the effectiveness of two types of speech re-education for functional articulation defectives as measured in terms of sound production and auditory discrimination for speech sounds. Ph.D. dissertation, New York University, 1959.

Shelton, R. L., *et al.:* A task for evaluation of articulation change: II.

Comparison of task scores during baseline and lesson series testing. J Speech Hear Res, 10:578-585, 1967.

Sommers, R. K. *et al.:* Training parents of children with functional misarticulation. J Speech Hear Res, 3:258-265, 1959.

Sommers, R. K., *et al.:* Effects of speech therapy and speech improvement upon articulation and reading. J Speech Hear Disord, 26:27-38, 1961.

Sommers, R. K., *et al.:* Effects of various durations of speech improvement upon articulation and reading. J Speech Hear Disord, 27:54-61, 1962a.

Sommers, R. K., *et al.:* Factors in the effectiveness of mothers trained to aid in speech correction. J Speech Hear Disord, 27:178-186, 1962b.

Sommers, R. K., *et al.:* The effectiveness of group and individual therapy. J Speech Hear Res, 9:219-255, 1966.

Sommers, R. K.: Problems in articulatory research: Methodology and error. ASHA, 9:406-408, 1967.

Sommers, R. K., *et al.:* Factors related to the effectiveness of articulation therapy for kindergarten, first and second grade children. J Speech Hear Res, 10:428-437, 1967.

Sommers, R. K., *et al.:* Factors in the effectiveness of articulation therapy with educable retarded children. J Speech Hear Res, 13:304-317, 1970.

Tufts, L. C., and Holliday, A. R.: Effectiveness of trained parents as speech therapists. J Speech Hear Disord, 24:395-401, 1959.

Van Riper, C., and Erickson, R.: A predictive screening test of articulation. J Speech Hear Disord, 34:214-219, 1969.

Ventura, R. P., Ingebo, G., and Wolmut, P.: A comparative evaluation of speech correction techniques in the primary grades and the role of maturation on misarticulation. ASHA, 2:378, 1960.

Weaver, J. B., and Wollersheim, J. P.: A comparison of the block system of scheduling speech cases in the public schools. ASHA, 6:392, 1964.

Webb, C., and Siegenthaler, B.: Comparison of aural stimulation methods for teaching speech sounds. J Speech Hear Disord, 22:264-270, 1957.

Wilson, B. A.: The development and evaluation of a speech improvement program for kindergarten children. J Speech Hear Disord, 19:4-13, 1954.

Winitz, H.: Articulatory Acquisition and Behavior. New York, Appleton-Century-Crofts, 1969.

Wood, K. S.: Parental maladjustment and functional articulation defects in children. J Speech Hear Disord, 11:255-275, 1946.

Wood, K. S.: The parent's role in the clinical program. J Speech Hear Disord, 13:209-210, 1948.

Wright, V., *et al.:* A task for evaluation of articulation change: III. Imitative task scores compared with scores for more spontaneous tasks. J Speech Hear Res, 12:875-884, 1969.

CHAPTER XI

AN ECLECTIC APPROACH TO
THE MANAGEMENT OF
ARTICULATION DISORDERS

ROBERT L. MILISEN

THE term eclectic, according to *Webster's Third Edition,* refers to a "selection which appears best from various diverse doctrines or methods." No doctrines, methods or theories have been reported that deal conclusively with differences in etiology, diagnosis and management of the articulation disorder. Many piece-meal differences, however, have been described and used. Clinicians approach the problem of defective articulation in vastly different ways and can usually state good reasons for their choice.

Some lean toward an organic explanation. They may blame deficiencies in the peripheral oral structures and/or the central nervous system for the disorder. Medical and dental treatment are often sought, and when these are ineffective, the client is given ear training and training in compensatory movements in an effort to overcome the structural and/or organic deficiency. These approaches tend to downgrade the importance of learning in the acquisition and maintenance of articulation skills.

Some clinicians believe that the problem can best be understood within the framework of linguistics. The assumption is made that the client has not followed the code that is standard for his culture. The method of treatment is to design models of primitive linguistic levels and build (through practice) toward the highest levels used in human communication. There is a tendency for such

233

an approach to become engrossed in linguistic structural concepts and to forget the importance of individual differences as they affect the disorder.

Some people believe the problem is rooted in some psychological disturbance in the client and that diagnosis and management of the disorder will depend on determining the nature of the maladjustment and ways of remedying it. There is a tendency for people who are interested in this approach to grant indulgence in organic and linguistic problems and to focus considerable attention upon individual differences.

More recently, attention has been devoted to the treatment of defective articulation as primarily a breakdown in the mechanics of learning. Treatment is often given with minimal attention to diagnosis since procedures are standardized and pre-programmed. This approach leans heavily on automated discrimination training. Any clinician who is trapped into using this as his whole approach must ignore most differences in the client's organic, environmental, psychological and learning backgrounds which may have influenced the client adversely.

Each of the above approaches may fit the needs of small groups of clients, but none of them are able to explain why *every* client has defective articulation nor how to modify the speech of *every* client until it meets the standards of his culture. Until these criteria are met, we will not have viable theories. For the time being, clinicians must consider an eclectic approach precisely because it is not possible to deal with articulation problems without giving attention to all conditions that have preceded onset or contributed to its development and maintenance. This means that all principles of science related to human growth and development must be focused on the problem if it is to be understood. It is painfully obvious that no book or collection of books has yet been written that covers all possible ramifications of the problem. The clinician must not, therefore, expect a text on speech pathology to cover the whole area. He must, instead, seek principles drawn from knowledge in such fields as physiology, psychology, genetics, linguistics, physics, mathematics and many others. Furthermore, no single book can cover all of the applied science information related to etiology, diagnosis and management of the articulation disorder. Accordingly, clinicians must study the application of scientific principles presented by writers dealing with disorders of learning, language and personality in order to obtain information which is relevant to the area of articulation.

This writer believes that therapy needs of articulation clients can be classified in two ways: (1) pre-behavioral therapy and (2) behavioral therapy. It would seem logical to discuss them in that sequence since a clinical program would deal with preparatory procedures before the actual therapy is initiated. However, in order to make the discussion as clear as possible for the reader, the sequence will be reversed, for the following reasons: (1) Pre-behavioral therapy includes such a broad spectrum of areas (most of which are the responsibility of other professions) that the reader may become lost in the multitude of options confronting him. (2) The choice of behavioral therapy is often dependent on a client's ability to react to its various phases. Consequently the clinician will be unable to appraise a client's needs until he understands the nature of behavioral therapy. (3) Most clients do not need pre-behavioral therapy.

CONCEPTS AFFECTING PRINCIPLES OF BEHAVIORAL ARTICULATION THERAPY

Several concepts must be understood before the clinician is qualified to plan and conduct this type of therapy. Many concepts have been measured empirically in clinical settings but not in strict laboratory environs. For this reason the reader must always be ready to question statements that are made and be prepared to adopt other alternatives. In the meantime, the following concepts will be used by the writer as the basis for solving articulation problems:

Concept 1. *Articulation, a type of learned behavior, is super-imposed on, and makes use of, physiological processes which are genetically determmined.*

Concept 2. *The learning process used in acquiring speech sounds is more complex than those used in developing most other skills requiring motor behavior.* This is due, in part, to the fact that the client has no way to objectively assess the similarity between his sound productions and those considered standard by his environment. He is usually dependent on an inverse process of self evaluation in which he is forced to depend on judgments of those around him in determining whether the way he produced a phoneme was right or wrong. By the age of 8 to 10 years, most children develop a skill of self evaluation and self regulation enabling them *automatically* to manipulate the way they articulate.

Concept 3. *The basis of behavioral therapy resides in "laws of learning."* The *laws* must be adapted in such a way as to allow the clinician and client to manipulate the client's speech behavior.

Concept 4. *The site of behavioral articulation therapy is found in speech situations in which the client participates.* The term *behavioral therapy* implies that rehabilitative processes must be focused on inter-behavior rather than on body structure or environment.

Since the act of initiating speech sounds must be learned and since this learning is dependent on cues fed back to the speaker following his attempts at communication, it is likely that the best schema for discussing behavioral articulation therapy is in a feedback model. Therapy may be focused on any phase of the feedback circuit. Usually clinicians focus on either the phase involving input into the client or the phase related to reinforcement of his output. Above all, however, clinicians must remember that they cannot change *one* part of the circuit without affecting *all* parts.

Two feedback circuits must be activated if communication between people is to develop. A third circuit which has considerable clinical value may be used in behavioral therapy. These three circuits are listed and discussed below.

Direct Circuit

This circuit has been called intra-personal, closed or internal. The term *closed* is poorly conceived and the term *internal* is confusing because some phases of this circuit are not found within the body. For instance, airborne vibrations of speech leave the speaker's mouth and return to his ear via air which is outside his body. This confusion could keep the person from understanding the clinical value of the third circuit, *indirect personal.*

The distinctive feature of the direct circuit is that the receptor organs that set it off are in the speaker and his speech response feeds back to his own receptor organs without help from any other person or any mechanical device.

Indirect Personal Circuit

This circuit has often been called inter-personal, external or relay. Two or more persons are needed to make this circuit possible since one must act as the speaker and another as the audience. The term *indirect* is descriptive of the circuit since the speaker's response does not come back directly to him but must be relayed to him through another person.

Indirect Impersonal Circuit

This circuit is usually omitted in feedback discussions. It is a circuit which involves indirect feedback cues since the speaker's response must be received by some impersonal device such as a mirror or tape-recorder and then be fed back to the speaker by the device. For the most part this circuit is not used by most children when learning to encode phonemes. Nonetheless, it could have facilitated such learning by objectifying the differences between their productions and standard patterns. Certainly this circuit is of great value to the clinician when making a diagnosis and when designing therapy for persons with defective articulation.

THERAPY PROCEDURES

The goal of management procedures is to help the client learn to modify his articulation productions in such a way that he produces all phonemes comfortably and spontaneously in all speech situations and in a manner accepted as standard by his culture.

Classification of Phoneme Errors

All encoding behavior involving phonemes may be placed into

two general groups for diagnostic and therapeutic purposes: (1) Unskilled responses that contain few elements of the standard phoneme. These responses may include complete omissions, substitutions of unrelated sounds (unvoicing of cognates would not represent this class) and severe distortions in which the physiological and acoustical characteristics used as representative of the phoneme deviate markedly from standard. Speech sounds in this group are consistently misarticulated by the client. (2) Partially skilled responses which contain some of the elements of the standard phoneme. These articulation responses include mild distortions and also sound substitution errors in which most of the acoustic characteristics are produced correctly as in substitutions of cognates. The client may also demonstrate inconsistent behavior in which the phoneme production may vary from "right" to "wrong." Inconsistent responses are a basic part of the learning process that occur prior to the time when standard responses are learned well enough to be habitual.

Relationship Between Unskilled and Partially Skilled Behavior

Principles and methods used by the client when learning to improve his articulation differ according to the level of skill he shows for each phoneme. For instance, the elimination of unskilled behavior usually begins with raw learning, sometimes accompanied by extinction learning and followed by transfer learning. Raw learning refers to the act of establishing a pattern where none existed previously. Transfer learning refers to the replacement of an incorrect pattern with a correct one. This act may require raw learning, but more often it depends on the transfer of skills learned in one situation to another situation where the client has not learned to use his skill. In addition, extinction learning may have to accompany transfer learning in order to eliminate persistently re-occurring faulty behavior.

Relationship Between Principles and Methods of Therapy

Principles refer to the rational basis used in choosing therapy processes. They are designed to show correlation between the problem to be dealt with and the rule or law that can be adapted or used in treating the problem. *Methods* are the specific clinical processes that have been chosen to solve the problem.

Whereas only one principle may be involved in solving a problem, a number of methods may be used, all of which may be effective in applying the principle. For example, what methods could be chosen to meet the following principle? "Acceptable articulation can be achieved only if the speaker can discriminate between his acceptable and unacceptable productions of speech sounds." Some of the methods that can be used to help the client achieve this skill are: (1) Have him listen to a recorded speech model, imitate it and evaluate his production for nearness of fit. Subsequently have him listen to the same model and then the tape recorded sample of his speech and ask him to reevaluate his phoneme for nearness of fit. (2) Have the client listen to a model spoken by the clinician, imitate the model and evaluate his imitation for nearness of fit. Compare his evaluation with that of the clinician. (3) Have the client listen and watch the clinician produce the model, imitate the model and evaluate it for nearness of fit. Have him repeat the process, but, in addition, have him pay special attention to the movements of the clinician's lips, jaw and tongue and then watch his own movements in a mirror while imitating the model. Subsequently he may appraise his imitation and compare it with his judgment of the speech production when he does not have objective feedback cues from the mirror.

Methods may be varied for many reasons, but usually it is because they have not produced the desired results or because the client has made enough progress and is ready to perform at a more advanced level.

Kinds of Management Needed by Persons with Defective Articulation

Needs differ with each client but three kinds of treatment may be indicated: (1) Psychotherapy is needed by some articulation defectives because the maladjustment is related to the quality of articulation or vice versa. This pre-behavioral therapy is closely related to motivation. (2) Organic treatment, either surgical, dental, prosthetic or medical, may also be needed by some persons. This pre-behavioral treatment may have a profound affect on articulation capacity if it is followed by behavioral therapy. (3) Behavioral manipulation is a type of management needed for the eradication of all types of *habitual* misarticulation even for those clients who need one or both of the other therapies.

While it is possible for many maladjusted or organically handicapped clients to acquire good articulation through the changes that can be achieved by behavioral manipulation alone, such a restricted clinical procedure is both unnecessarily difficult and time consuming. Consequently, for those persons whose maladjustment or organic condition is clearly related to their disorder of articulation, psychotherapy and/or organic treatment should either precede behavioral manipulation or occur concomitantly with it.

BEHAVIORAL ARTICULATION THERAPY

This type of therapy is always administered within a communication context of some kind. Its management, therefore, involves a careful manipulation of the various feedback systems between the speaker and other persons or between the speaker and various objective feedback systems.

A person's speech behavior can be manipulated by focusing on either of two phases of his communication act: the stimulus which sets off his speech response or the reinforcement of his encoded response. The stimulus will determine, to a degree, the nature of the succeeding response. The nature of the reinforcement of the speaker's response may affect the stability of many subsequent responses. One cannot assume when he focuses on the speaker's input and output systems that input refers exclusively to stimulus and output to reinforcement. Both stimulus and reinforcement affect the speaker only through his receptor system but involve different parts of his feedback circuits. Further explanation, therefore, is needed in distinguishing between these two kinds of therapy.

Stimulus model refers to the stimulus information (visual-acoustic-tactile), directed toward the speaker, which provides a speech pattern for the speaker to follow. It is the beginning of a circuit. Although this kind of model provides an important way of manipulating the person's speech, it is not as important as many clinicians believe. In fact, there are times when this type of therapy is a greater handicap than a help. For this reason, the clinician must be sure he understands the principles behind every therapy process involving stimulus models.

Response reinforcement refers to the nature of our reaction to the speaker's speech and the manner used in stimulating his receptor organs after he has spoken. It is a reinforcement which closes the feedback circuit. Positive reinforcement of the manner of articulation can be achieved by stimulating the client's receptors by either words or gestures that convey approval. This reward can be directed toward the manner of articulation ("That's good.") or to the content ("I understand."). Negative reinforcement can be given by specific rejection of the manner of production ("That sound wasn't right.") or by misunderstanding speech ("What did you say?"). All types of reinforcement will reach the client only through his receptors and, according to the theory of inverse process of self evaluation, will be a primary determiner in the shaping of subsequent sounds and their maintenance *regardless of closeness of fit between the phoneme as produced and the environmental standard.*

PRINCIPLES OF THERAPY INVOLVING MODEL STIMULATION

This type of therapy is significant only if the stimulation reaches the client and sets off a response. Its effectiveness may be explained in one of two ways. Mowrer (1950) proposed the possibility that the young imitate those whom they love and in whose footsteps they wish to follow. He used imitative behavior of birds partially as a support of this concept. In a sense, this implies that the infant learns to initiate a new and unfamiliar kind of behavior by imitating the stimulator.

A different rationale grows out of the assumption that nothing new is created in the universe or in man's behavior. Every movement in the universe and every activity of man has its antecedents in previous movements and activities. If antecedent conditions are identified and understood, subsequent behavior can be predicted and controlled. Insofar as model stimulation therapy is concerned, the rationale asserts that no new movement is produced by the child. Rather, the stimulus activates a circuit which had previously been used (albeit in performance of a different purpose). For example, sucking is a *wired-in* physiological process for most infants. The tongue is pressed against the nipple which in turn is pressed against the alveolar ridge. Sometimes the movement of the tongue is pushed directly against the ridge (either when the nipple is removed, or while the infant is preparing to suck). These movements of the tongue and the accompanying closure of the velo-pharyngeal port are similar to the ones that are used in producing the /t/ and /d/ phonemes. Speech stimulation may re-activate this circuit but for a different purpose than sucking.

The concept that all speech movements have their antecedents in primitive movements can be tested easily with animals and humans. People working with porpoises have tried to teach them to talk. They have used human speech as their stimuli and have had little success, largely because they have insisted in trying to teach the porpoise to perform a task (humanoid sounds) that is entirely new to him. Yet there is much evidence that porpoises do communicate with each other by using clicks and whistles which are easy for them to make from their blow hole. It is quite possible that the human could develop a code to use with the porpoise, if he used the sounds commonly produced by that animal. Dogs can be trained to reproduce many movements and sounds, so long as one builds on skills previously used. The writer's dog, Arf, can be caused to produce a sneeze-like sound if stimulated with a loudly exploded fricative /f/ sound. In the beginning, this was not possible unless the stimulus was given immediately after she sneezed. Her stimulated sneeze could be elicited for longer and longer periods of time after the real sneeze had occurred. The time came when the stimulus elicited the simulated behavior without being preceded by a real sneeze. This kind of conditioning has been amply described in many experiments reported by Skinner (1957). Some people have referred to the revival of previously used skills as the re-activation of reverberating circuits. Obviously a circuit cannot be re-activated until it has been closed. Once closed, it may be transferred into many settings provided conditioning methods are used which will enable the client to initiate or retrieve the circuit independently of physiological conditions which caused it to emerge initially.

The following principles of model stimulation therapy are based on the assumption that stimuli designed to elicit encoding responses are effective only if they activate circuits that have been used previously. The chief purpose of model stimulation is to narrow the range of response patterns so the clinician will have more encoded behavior of a specific nature to manipulate.

Operant conditioning procedures directed toward random behavior arising from non-specific stimuli waste time of the clinician because he must wait for long periods of time before the client produces the desired encoded response. The smaller the number of responses that can be reinforced in a given period of time, the slower the learning. This can be checked experimentally in many ways. Greenspoon (1955) measured the effect of reinforcement on word choice. His experimental procedure required subjects to produce words singly and in meaningless order. He reinforced only the plural nouns and, of course, most subjects produced very few plural nouns during the first part of the experiment since they had been given no specific instruction to narrow their choice. If this same method were used by a clinician who wishes to work on the /θ/ sound, it may be necessary to wait while hundreds of phonemes are produced by his client before one /θ/ phoneme will occur spontaneously. This trial-and-error method can be eliminated by presenting a stimulus for a specific response that has been produced previously. The model used for the /θ/ might involve the protrusion of the tongue between the teeth, a stimulus that can be seen as well as heard. It is a movement that is quite similar to tongue movements made by most clients from infancy.

With the assumption that stimulus models narrow the field of response behavior as well as activating previously used circuits for a different purpose, let us consider the different principles involved in using stimulus models in behavioral therapy.

(1) *The client must be able to discriminate the stimulus model from other stimuli before it will effectively directionalize his response pattern.* Deaf children may not be able to discriminate between acoustic stimuli. Deaf-blind children will not discriminate between acoustic and visual stimuli. Autistic children may not discriminate stimuli composed of acoustic, visual and tactile stimuli and yet under certain conditions, when suitable stimuli are given in an appropriate setting, these children may discriminate very effectively.

(2) *The client must be receptive to the stimulus model before it will effectively influence his behavior.* Meaningless stimuli will often fall on "deaf" ears. Sounds that are of no consequence, as far as the child is concerned, are not likely to move him to action. Receptivity for models not only implies a compatibility between the clinician and his client but also the purpose of the stimulus model as conceived by the clinician and the client. If it is intended as a way of modifying the client's speech pattern, the stimulus goal is intended to elicit sounds and movements, not speech and language. If, on the other hand, the goal is speech communication, the stimulus model will be secondary to communication and will become a non-specific way of eliciting articulation. Non-specific models are less likely to be effective than specific ones.

(3) *Stimulus models presented in a clear and vivid manner are more effective than those that are not.* For instance, phonemes produced through clenched teeth or mumbled are not likely to be effective. Phonemes that are presented so the client can see the movements used in making them, as well as hear them distinctly, will be more vivid. Sometimes tactile stimulation will also add to the vividness.

(4) *Stimulus models will be more effective if they replicate some behavior for which the client has had some recent experience.* The babbling sounds made by an infant are more likely to be induced by stimulation that follows shortly after the infant has finished babbling than if a longer time elapses. In a sense this is one of the results achieved by Froeschels (1932) when he had his clients talk while chewing.

(5) *Stimulus models will be more effective if the maturity of the speech patterns used is comparable to the client's competence.*

Sounds in isolation are unacceptable stimulus models for the client who is able to produce them in syllables. Sounds in syllables as models are unacceptable if the client is able to say them in words. In the same way, language models involving first grade level concepts in first grade language forms are unacceptable for clients who can function at an adult level of grammar and vocabulary.

(6) *Stimulus models will be more effective if the client is able to make objective comparisons between the model he received and the response he makes.* A client may not have a precise way of judging the adequacy of his response to a model stimulus. Therefore, he must depend on feedback from some source outside of himself. Usually the feedback comes from people. This is quite unsatisfactory since the assessments of the speech responses may be inaccurate or misleading. Moreover, the client may find it impossible to determine whether the responses elicited are to the quality of his articulation or to his speech content. Thus the client does not know whether his articulation was good or poor when he depends on reinforcements made by people. (Many defective-speaking college students are shocked when told they have defective articulation because they had never been made aware of their deficiency.) A variety of feedback systems that are simultaneous (mirror) or delayed (tape-recorder, video tape) give the client a means of objectifying his response with the stimulus model and thereby circumventing the inconsistencies and obtuseness of subjective reinforcements.

PRINCIPLES OF THERAPY INVOLVING REINFORCEMENT

Reinforcement given to the client after he produces a phoneme may take a variety of forms. It may be specific or general and/or subjective or objective. *Specific* reinforcement is any reaction to the *process* of articulation, not the *content* of language, and is designed to control or manipulate articulation. ("That was a good sound.") *General* reinforcement is any reaction to spoken language which is directed to *content* of language, not to *process* of articulation but one which will, nevertheless, influence the nature of articulation. ("Oh, I see what you mean.") *Subjective* reinforcements will be given by members of the audience and may be either specific or general as illustrated above. They have the weakness of imposing on the speaker all of the biases and inconsistencies of the listener. *Objective* reinforcements are almost always specific to the process of articulation. They result from an interaction between the speaker and some objective feedback system that allows him to compare objectively his production of a phoneme with standard production of the same phoneme.

With the assumption that reinforcement of human behavior exerts a powerful influence on the maintenance of some behavioral patterns and the eradication of others, let us consider some of the principles governing this important clinical tool as they influence the design of behavioral therapy.

(1) *Any condition, occurring during or after the production of a phoneme, that affects subsequent productions of that phoneme must be considered a form of reinforcement.* Many clinicians and parents assume that reactions to the client's speech must be specifically directed to the production of the phoneme if a client's speech is to be improved. Conversely, they believe that statements made in an off-hand manner do not provide reinforcement. Of course both assumptions are incorrect and unfortunately result in the loss of opportunity to facilitate good speech patterns on the one hand or cause the retention of faulty ones on the other.

(2) *The shorter the lapse of time between the response and its reinforcement, the stronger the effect on learning.* Every speech event is loaded with variables, and the number increases rapidly as a function of time. The greater the number of variables involved, the greater the probability that the influence of reinforcement will be diluted because many reinforcements will be associated with the wrong variable. The playing back of a recorded sample of phonemes after a lapse of three or four minutes of speech will be much less effective as a therapy measure than if played back immediately. During the long lapse of time, the client has had many additional experiences, and the memory of the physiological processes used in making the sound will have dimmed before he receives the feedback, thus increasing the chance that he will associate the reinforcement with the wrong process.

(3) *The more validly the reinforcement relates to the quality of the speech response, the more effective it will be.* Reinforcement

schedules which result in both positive and negative reactions to similar productions of a phoneme will result in confusion on the part of the client and will produce inconsistent behavior. This kind of inconsistency is, unfortunately, the lot of all children during the period in which speech is being developed. Parents are confronted with conflicting goals; they want to understand what their child says, and at the same time they want their child to speak clearly. If a child's speech is intelligible but contains many misarticulations, the parent is forced to make a decision. Should he respond by reacting to what the child said, or should he ignore meaning of speech and react to how the child articulated? If he follows the first procedure he will reinforce *positively* his child's misarticulations. If instead, he ignores meaning and reacts to articulation ("You didn't make that sound right."), he is likely to interfere with the development of language as a medium of communication.

(4) *The more frequently a phoneme is reinforced validly, provided it is produced correctly part of the time, the greater will be the probability that subsequent productions will resemble a standard pattern.* The greater the number of reinforcements (both positive and negative) that are received by the client for his articulation, the more opportunities he has to compare the physiological processes he used in producing correct sounds with those he used when producing them incorrectly. The more comparisons he can make, the sooner he will be able to self-regulate with accuracy those processes he needs to use in producing the phoneme in a standard manner.

(5) *Reinforcement of deviant productions of a particular phoneme will manipulate successive productions in the direction of normal if paired responses are rewarded differentially.* A client who is unable to produce all characteristics of a phoneme but who varies his production from time to time can be moved toward standard speech by rewarding successive approximations, i.e. by reinforcing the best of a series of responses. For example, a child who has trouble closing his lips may be rewarded when lips more nearly approximate on one attempt than on another by "That last one was better than the other."

(6) *Speech behavior can be modified by giving only positive*

reinforcement to the good productions and ignoring all others. In the beginning, this type of reinforcement is the safest to use because it draws attention only to the successful performances. This experience usually will not disturb the client. If the habit is not too deep-seated the behavior pattern will change since the *body computer* is able to separate suitable physiological patterns from the unacceptable ones and to facilitate his self-regulation until most of his error responses are eliminated.

(7) *Reinforcement of speech behavior will produce more stable patterns if only some of the good productions are reinforced rather than all of them.* During the early stages in training, a client will be able to change his speech behavior more rapidly if every good production is rewarded. If, however, this schedule of hundred per cent reinforcement continues, the client begins to expect it every time he articulates correctly. Obviously this type of reinforcement schedule cannot always be maintained during speech. Nevertheless, if the client has come to expect positive reinforcement for each good response, he may look upon all responses that are not rewarded as failures. This worry about unreinforced normal phonemes may cause him to change them the next time he talks.

(8) *The more exactly the reinforcement helps the client identify good phoneme characteristics from poor ones, the more readily he will be able to adopt those that are good and extinguish the others.* Since the client does not recognize the nature of his own speech error (inverse process of self-evaluation) he is greatly assisted if the reinforcement is of such a nature that he can see precisely the difference between his error production and the standard. For example, some clients have the ability to close the velo-pharyngeal port but do not do so while speaking. His plosives and fricatives are accompanied by a great deal of nasal air emission. Nasal olives and candle flame will demonstrate the difference between the client's breath pattern and that used by other people. Continued use of this device will enable him to learn to close the port if he pays attention to differential amounts of air coming from the nose while producing sounds successively. He can now transfer his appropriate movements (velo-pharyngeal closure) to sounds which previously had nasal air emission. It is important

to note that most of these changes will take place without the client being able to tell how the change came about.

(9) *Self-controlled reinforcements coming from the indirect impersonal circuit are less threatening to the client than those given by a clinician in an indirect subjective circuit.* The client who can use a mechanical device (tape-recorder, mirror, nasal olives, etc.) as a means of becoming acquainted with his anomalous behavior and of modifying it will be under less strain than if he has to depend on a person for his source of evaluation and reinforcement. This is true even if the client is very fond of the other person. In fact, the more he likes the other person the more disturbed he may be when he continues to make a mistake, whereas alone with the tape-recorder, he can try to make the sound over and over again without feelings of shame.

(10) *Reinforcements provided by indirect impersonal circuits must be carefully programmed so error and correct responses are not confused by the client.* Since the maintenance or extinction of a behavior pattern depends on the client's impression of which of his physiological patterns were correct and which ones were not, it is obvious that the clinical task must be so arranged that he will not be able to obtain a false impression. The machine cannot correct his errors in interpretation, but the clinician can before the client tries to perform the task independently. For example, one child with repaired cleft palate was trying to learn to direct air out of the mouth and not the nose. A set of nasal olives was used as the mechanical device. She reported success in producing a number of her difficult sounds without nasal emission. Careful inspection of the olives indicated that the holes into the olives were covered with tissue in the nares. As a result air could not pass through them, and they in turn closed the nasal passage. Although it was true that the child did not have nasal air emission, her success, unfortunately, was due to faulty programming of the task, not to a newly learned skill. The clinician should have protected against this error by having the child inhale and exhale air through the nose while the nasal olives were in place. Failure of air to pass through them would have given evidence that the device was defective and that the client would receive faulty reinforcement from it.

(11) *Negative effects from a faulty articulation habit will cause the extinction of the habit provided (1) the client can make the standard response part of the time and (2) he identifies the times when he does not produce it correctly.* Facial tics, persistent word errors in typing, misarticulations, etc., can, under special circumstances, be eliminated by practicing them *voluntarily.* Without this practice or without some other therapy process, well established habits may last a life time. The client's level of motivation must be high and the goals of negative practice thoroughly understood, otherwise the practice of the faulty pattern is likely to strengthen rather than extinguish the bad habit.

The rationale for negative practice is that cues from the client's behavior feed back to him, making him aware of certain movements which had previously been produced automatically and subliminally. The person penalizes himself every time he voluntarily makes himself produce the error response. In a sense he says to himself, "I wish I didn't make this error; I must try not to do it in the future when I talk." The more he practices the error, the more sensitive he is to the feedback cues. The sooner he can identify each error response that begins automatically, the sooner he will be able to stop it and to replace it with a correct one. As a result of this sequence he develops a skill of self-regulation that enables him to automatically and spontaneously produce the correct speech response without being aware of the process that is taking place.

PRINCIPLES OF THERAPY INVOLVING DISCRIMINATION

This type of therapy has been the storm center of considerable professional controversy. Some speech pathologists routinely prescribe a traditional type of *ear training* as a part of every articulation program. These traditional discrimination practices require the client to distinguish between sounds produced by the clinician. The client may be stimulated by sounds composed of phonemes, as well as by non-speech sounds such as ringing of bells, piano tones, etc. The theoretical basis for such practices is that etiology of articulation grows out of an inability to distinguish between speech sounds and that this weakness leads to faulty imitations, i.e. misarticulation.

Another type of discrimination training that is gaining recognition involves the client's perception of his own speech sound productions and through processes of self-evaluation to compare them with standards set by his environment.

Succeeding principles of discrimination therapy discussed in this chapter are based on the belief that promiscuous training of discrimination at the least is wasteful of time and at the worst harmful to the client. The clinician may not feel the need to program specific methods to meet the needs of the client and the client may be bored with the infantile practices that are required of him. However, appropriate discrimination training which is designed to overcome inadequacies that are distinctive to each client is a prerequisite for his improvement.

(1) *Traditional (decoding) ear training is needed by clients who are unable to understand speech composed of linguistic units adapted to his age and ability.* Many persons cannot decode phonemes, words, phrases or sentences spoken in a normal manner. This deficiency has a detrimental effect on both the decoding and encoding process and deserves careful clinical planning. In addition, many persons have difficulty, according to test scores, in discriminating between various speech sounds presented in highly artificial conditions. It is doubtful that this apparent deficiency warrants intensive clinical treatment, provided the client can discriminate these phonemes and syllables and use them effectively in decoding meaningful speech. Certainly our goal is not to teach skill in discrimination under highly artificial conditions. The goal is, instead, to train the client to discriminate in such a way that it will help him articulate his phonemes in an acceptable manner.

(2) *Many people who fail traditional discrimination tests should not be given traditional ear training.* Many persons who fail the traditional discrimination tests do so because of the inadequacy of the test measure rather than because of an inability to use discrimination for speech purposes. Hit and miss discrimination training for these people is a waste of time and can serve to destroy motivation. We are not trying to improve discrimination but rather articulation. Two good methods are available to

clinicians in determining whether decoding discrimination training is needed: (1) Determine if the client can be stimulated with the sound. If he can produce it correctly, it is doubtful that decoding ear training is needed. (2) Study in depth the ability of the person to distinguish between his error sound and other sounds that have similar characteristics. If he has trouble, then ear training, *specific to that phoneme,* may be needed.

(3) *Ear training that appears to activate the decoding circuit may be effective for clients who can produce a phoneme correctly part of the time, if the training also activates the encoding discrimination circuit.* One of the tenets of clinical practice is to enable the client to become involved with his own improvement. Tasks that require the client to make judgments may be helpful if those judgments are accompanied with action. While a client listens to speech, he also experiences some empathic responses (subliminal speech imitations). Discriminations that activate one of the client's faulty circuits and help him compare it to an appropriate one are likely to precipitate improvement, *provided the client has learned to produce that phoneme correctly part of the time.*

(4) *Self-evaluative (encoding) discrimination is more closely related to the articulation process used in encoding linguistic patterns than discrimination of another's utterances.* Discrimination used in linguistic coding is composed of two closely related but nevertheless independent variables. Practice in one form of discrimination will not necessarily affect improvement in the other, unless it involves an overlapping of both the encoding and decoding processes, as illustrated in the previous principle that was just described. Ear training involving discrimination is more closely related to manipulation of articulation behavior and can occur only during the time the client is speaking or immediately after he has finished. His act of comparing his phonemic productions with standards set by his environment will, if they are valid comparisons, have a powerful effect on extinguishing his misarticulations and strengthening his standard ones. On the other hand, if his self-evaluations are invalid, he is likely to make few changes, or if they are made, they are not likely to be unrelated to standard speech.

(5) *Skillful encoding discrimination is essential to the acquisition of standard articulation, but usually it is learned incidentally through association processes rather than through intentional conditioning processes.* The child does not try, for the most part, to learn to articulate as his environment articulates. He tries, instead, to behave in a manner that will obtain for him the cooperation of his environment. Gestures and signals such as crying are inefficient methods of communication. Gradually as he matures and produces many movements and sounds, he learns that some physiological processes are more frequently associated in the resolution of his problems than others, i.e. his family does something for him while he cries but is not likely to respond to him when he wiggles his toes. Through this associative process, the cry becomes conditioned to need-reduction, and he begins to evoke the cry when he has a need. One might say that an intentional act of communication grew out of many experiences in which certain physiological acts were incidentally associated with need-reduction. It is not possible for him to develop specific acts of communication until he has learned that some of his *reflex* responses manipulate his audience more effectively than others. It is proposed that the same kind of incidental conditioning of physiological processes converts them into movements of speech which the child is able to evoke when needed.

PRINCIPLES OF PRE-ARTICULATION THERAPY

The capacities and performances of the client will determine the nature of the therapy pattern. Since behavioral articulation therapy should not be introduced unless the client is capable of decoding speech, even though defectively, it is obvious that pre-articulation therapy may require basic attention to a variety of conditions, such as organic impairment and environmental deterrents to speech development, and to the status of communication skills which are prerequisite to speech. This therapy covers such a wide range of services and treatments that the best that can be offered in this discussion is a direction for attacking the problem rather than a specific methodology.

Organic Disabilities

For organically handicapped children who are delayed in development of linquistic communication skills, the therapy goals require services of many professions. Required frequently are services ranging from medical and surgical to prosthetic intervention. No progression of treatment can be stated for the organically handicapped because each has his own problems, and each problem must be solved by a well trained professional. However, a rule can be stated: The earlier in the child's life that correction or compensation is achieved, the better the chances are that the child will develop normal articulation.

Principles of Management of Organic Deviations: A Type of Pre-Behavioral Therapy

There is no perfect speech mechanism just as there is no perfect phonemic pattern. Each person, while learning to manipulate his movements in order to produce phonemes that will serve as a part of a linguistic code, must control his imperfect speech mechanism so it will produce speech sounds in a manner expected by his audience. The greater the mechanism deviates from a mythically perfect one, the greater the barrier to standard behavior.

Organic deviations of the peripheral-oral structures and/or the structures of the central nervous system are of prime concern to the speech pathologist and audiologist. The causes of these deviations may be inherited or acquired before or after birth.

A special type of organic deviation that is usually not considered but may, nevertheless, have a profound effect on the nature of articulation is one that is acquired as a residue of experience. The whole body, and particularly the nervous system, goes through subtle changes during the time while learning is developing. Whether this change results from a deposit in the neural tissues called engrams or some kind of chemical change in a whole neural feedback circuit that leads to *reverberating circuits,* the fact remains that the organism is different after the experience than it was before. These acquired organic conditions undoubtedly contribute to the rigidity or irreversibility of various learned behavior patterns.

Regardless of the nature of the organic deviations that are present, the clinician must consider them in designing his management program. The disadvantages arising from organic deviations may be dealt with in various ways. Some structural anomalies involving the ear, palate, teeth and lip may be surgically repaired. Others must be compensated for by artificial media such as hearing aids and dental obturators, by medicines or by clinical procedures that either strengthen tissues or train others to assume new functions. The clinician must be careful not to diagnose a disorder as having *no organic involvement* if the client's faulty speech behavior is *habitual* or highly consistent.

Regardless of the kind of organic involvement that is present (and some is probably always present), the clinician must make allowance for it in his management design. Some of the principles that will guide him in this design are:

(1) *Structural disorders should be corrected (when possible) before speech is developed.* If speech habits develop which incorporate the disordered tissue, not only will the surrounding tissues orient to the anomaly and become an established part of the faulty behavior, but also engrams or reverberating circuits will be built up that will resist changes when clinical training is administered.

(2) *No organic deviation, whether structural or otherwise, will determine independently the end-product of phonemic encoding. However, compensatory procedures are to be indicated when the anomaly cannot be corrected.* Some deaf people learn to understand speech and some can encode it with clarity. Many people with dental, palatal, lingual and laryngeal disorders acquire good articulation and voice in spite of the physical handicap. But their learning may have been implemented by medical or dental care or by prosthetic therapy.

(3) *If compensatory procedures are indicated in the therapy design, the earlier they begin (before habitual patterns of speech become deep-seated), the greater the chance they will be effective.* Oral language training of deaf children will be many times more effective if it is begun at one year of age than at six. Children with unrepaired cleft palates can more often learn to talk with little

audible abnormality if the training begins early (six months) than if it begins at six years. In fact, little difference from *normal* children's language and articulation development will be observed if surgery is finished before one year of age.

PRINCIPLES OF MANAGEMENT INVOLVING MOTIVATION: A TYPE OF PRE-BEHAVIORAL THERAPY

Very few people with defective articulation lack the capacity to improve their speech. Unfortunately, however, many of them do not show improvement even with the help of highly skilled clinicians. Great capacity of a client to learn and excellent skills of the clinician can be nullified by poor motivation. Some clients are simply uninterested while other are openly hostile. To insist on conducting behavioral articulation therapy for the uninterested person is, at the least, a waste of time, and for the hostile individual, therapy is often harmful.

It is often difficult for young clinicians to believe that a person with a handicap would not welcome the chance to correct it. Unfortunately, this is not the case. More time is spent preparing some clients to be receptive to therapy than is spent on articulation therapy itself. The fact that many handicapped people actively resist opportunities to improve is not so difficult to understand if one considers that once a behavior has become learned, it is more comfortable to continue it unchanged. Furthermore, people become identified with all aspects of their behavior and to change them would seem "artificial" and inconsistent with their self concepts.

Motivation which will implement therapy must grow out of a client's belief that he needs to change his speech, that a change is possible and that a change will be pleasant and advantageous. The clinician can be helpful only if he is honest and realistic in all his interpersonal behavior with the client. He must be honest with himself also. He must face the fact that a person typically initiates only that kind of behavior which is to his advantage. At the same time the clinician must also recognize that no one, including himself, can take care of his own needs independently. Each person is dependent on other people for the solution of practically every problem.

How do these concepts about motivation relate to a client who is either uninterested or hostile to clinical work? First of all the client, whether young or old, must be helped to understand the end product of continuing in the same direction. Second, the clinician must not cling to the idea that he is being generous and doing everything for the client and nothing for himself. He must admit openly that he is receiving advantages too. This helps to eliminate the "holier than thou" attitude and makes clinical services easier to accept by many clients.

Another matter that needs early attention is the demonstration of the fact that speech can be improved. Many clients pretend disinterest because they have been disappointed by the results of therapy so many times and may have been criticized unfairly after they tried and failed. They do not intend to be backed into another *clinical corner.* An opportunity to observe other people with similar problems and to objectively observe themselves is often helpful. It is especially useful to let the client carry on a dialogue with other persons who have the same kind of problem. Discussions of this kind can melt icy negativism or dissolve studied indifference and prepare the way for a willingness to try. Motivation, when it comes, means that the client is ready to take a chance on succeeding even though this willingness to try leaves him open to risks of discouragement and failure.

Faulty motivation is not a burden to be borne by the client alone. Responsibility for it must also be carried by counterfeit clinicians, uninterested or aggressive parents and part of the time by honest clinicians who have used counterfeit practices. Such practices refer to any method used in a clinical session that is not specifically designed to alleviate the client's problem. *Cookbook recipes,* such as "spend the first part of each session on ear training and follow that with stimulation of the phoneme in isolation" or "I always find that it helps the child to bite down on his lip," are a detriment to progress since they prescribe practices indiscriminately. Even worse are the games to which so many clinicians are addicted. These games not only waste time because they are not specifically related to the problem, but they say to the client loud and clear, "I know you don't want to face your articulation problems and work objectively toward their eradication, but maybe you can be tricked into improvement by playing games; at least you won't complain about coming to therapy class." Often the counterfeit clinician is as poorly motivated to conduct a clinical session as the hostile client is to participate in it.

The following principles of therapy, where motivation is the primary concern, are based on the belief that behavioral articulation therapy directed toward a poorly motivated client is a waste of time; and, therefore, the matter of motivations must be the first concern of the clinician if the client is uninterested or hostile toward rehabilitation. A good diagnosis should evaluate the attitude of the client and his family toward rehabilitation.

(1) *Therapy can begin immediately if the client and his family have a high level of motivation for rehabilitation.* Some clients and their families are eager for help. With these people, the goal is to design the program in such a way that success can be demonstrated often enough to keep the interest high. It is important that all participants receive some reward for earlier behavior that has contributed to the good attitude, ("The way you helped him at home was marvelous.") Everyone must continue to participate and be rewarded as the therapy progresses.

(2) *Articulation therapy cannot begin for clients who are uninterested because they are unaware of the difference in their speech and its importance to their future.* Usually these clients and their family need objective evidence of the presence of a disorder and its implications for the person's future. (One mother would not believe her fifteen-year-old, cleft-palate daughter had speech that was largely unintelligible to strangers until it was demonstrated to her that she was unable to interpret the daughter's tape-recorded speech.) With such people, suitable motivation levels may be reached as soon as they are convinced that a problem does exist and that methods are available for its treatment.

(3) *Articulation therapy cannot begin for some clients because either they or their family are uninterested.* When a high enough motivation level is present for the family but not for the client, the clinician must find ways of showing the client the advantages he will receive from improved speech. Sometimes the client is motivated, but the family is not. This disinterest may be due to many reasons. Sometimes adults think the child will outgrow the

disorder. In this case discussions about developmental levels of speech performance may be helpful especially if examples of developmental arrest are described. Sometimes parents believe the child is unable to make improvement and that the best way of coping is to ignore the problem and to learn to accept it. Two-way mirrors provide parents with excellent means for judging the accuracy of their observations without having to be in front of the child. The clinician may change a parental point of view by demonstrating a technique of therapy which brings immediate improvement for the child.

Sometimes deep-seated personality problems interfere with acceptance of the presence of the disorder. In this case the clinician should refer the client to a psychotherapist or psychiatrist.

(4) *Articulation therapy cannot begin for clients who are hostile to it.* Therapy programs will be sabotaged by persons who are hostile to them. The first task for the clinician is to determine the basis for the hostility and to correct for it before introducing articulation therapy.

In some instances the problem is fairly apparent. Sometimes the client has been subjected to poor clinical services and has become skeptical of all similar services. Sometimes the resistance is an outgrowth of too much pressure from home or community. In either instance, objective discussions and demonstrations to the client and family may straighten out the problem. If the attitude has a deeper personality base, psychotherapy will be needed. In any event the resistance should be reduced before behavioral articulation therapy begins.

Environmental Deficiencies

For the child whose life is being devastated by a bad environment, the task may be difficult to deal with because the evidence is not as easy to isolate as in the case of organic disabilities. In addition, remedial procedures are less specific or may not be available in any form. Children in orphanges, children living in their natural homes with parents who do not want them and children in hospitals where they are a statistic on a chart may receive little or no love and attention, which are essential if communication skills are to be learned.

A variety of changes may be possible. Sometimes a complete change is achieved by finding a new home for the child. Sometimes the adults have been confused as to the manner to be used in handling the child and are willing and anxious to modify their behavior and to follow suggestions. Sometimes new people can be inserted into the environment to ameliorate a bad situation to a degree, or the child may be sent to visit Aunt Martha for a couple of weeks while the parents are on vacation. Unfortunately, agencies too often have neither the money nor the trained personnel to cope with problems of their public charges. Many parents are unwilling to accept any responsibility for the child's failures or to change their lives in ways which would create a better environment for the child.

For children who are delayed in developing communication skills, the following principles of communication therapy of a pre-linguistic nature may be employed:

(1) *Begin at the level where the child is performing.* Some children have either been ignored or rejected and, as a result, have not had an opportunity to acquire a medium for communicating with their environment. Many of these children do not use the cry to signal their needs, but they often whine intermitantly. They wait to be cared for, and they do not assert their wishes and needs in any consistent way. The overt physiological responses of these children have either been totally ignored by their environment, or the child is so handicapped sensorially that the people around him cannot make contact.

(2) *The level at which therapy must begin for some children involves the creation of a rudimentary non-verbal communication pattern the child can use in manipulating his environment.* Usually this involves the conditioning of certain types of behavior produced by the client which precede or occur concomitantly with various needs. Sounds, grimaces or any other behavior that is related to the child's needs can be reinforced by solving the child's needs. The goal of this therapy is achieved when the child initiates this kind of behavior more often and more persistently before or during the time when his needs arise.

(3) *A higher therapy level may be needed by children who are ready to initiate sounds and movements without a physiological setting and primary reinforcers.* The child is ready for advancement as soon as he has become aware of his environment and has successfully manipulated it by initiating smiles, cries and other non-verbal behavior. He must learn to convert various involuntary physiological movements into events that he can initiate voluntarily. For instance, he must learn to initiate sounds and noises, some of which will be closely related to phonemes of speech. The end goal of these voluntary acts as far as the child is concerned may be self entertainment or a means of attracting attention. Two theoretical concepts have a bearing on the manner whereby this skill develops. One might be called the *theory of mimicry.* It states that the child learns by imitating the sounds of other people. A special interpretation of this concept is suggested by Mowrer (1950), who believes the child does this because he wishes to be like his love object. The other theory might be called *transference.* This requires the conversion of movements serving a purpose to movements used in the language code through conditioning processes. This concept insists that the child has already experienced most of the movements involved in producing phonemes. The chief task involves conditioning of his behavior so he can initiate a sound rather than waiting for it to occur more or less reflexly.

(4) *Another therapy level is designed to create understanding between the child and his environment so the child will decode speech and perform simple non-linguistic responses.* If linguistic behavior is to become the primary communication tool of the child, he must learn to understand it when spoken by other people. Since it is easier for him to decode than encode speech, learning to understand speech would be given precedence over learning to speak it, at least in the early period of his life.

(5) *The highest level of pre-articulation therapy is directed toward motivating the child to encode words as a medium of communication.* The speech model stimulus given by the adult is composed of only a few of the sounds the child is capable of producing. This will tend to constrain the selection of sounds by the child. If this constraint does not occur, the child is likely to

encode a foreign type of speech which will have little communication value. A further constraint is provided by the listener when he reinforces *words* containing some sounds and ignores others. Nevertheless, any speech attempt, especially at the beginning of speech development, should be attended to and reinforced in such a way as to encourage the child to produce a larger number of responses which will be available for manipulation and modification by the clinician.

CONCLUSION

The goal of an eclectic approach to the management of defective articulation is to provide every client with the skills needed to produce speech sounds at levels accepted as standard by his culture. The principles and methods to be used in accomplishing this goal may be drawn from many academic and service areas so long as they serve the needs of the client. The participation of the clinician will be both scientific and artistic; he must solve problems like a scientist and he must accomplish his task with the feeling of an artist. Above all, the clinician must be professional enough to give service only when he is qualified and to seek assistance when the needs of his clients over-reach the level of his competence.

REFERENCES

Froeschels, E.: Infant Speech. Boston, Expression Company, 1932.
Greenspoon, J.: The reinforcement effect of two spoken sounds on the frequency of two responses. Am J Psychol, 68:409-416, 1955.
Mowrer, O. H.: Learning Theory and Personality Dynamics. New York, Ronald Press Co. 1950.
Skinner, B. F.: Verbal Behavior. New York, Appleton-Century-Crofts, 1957.

AUTHOR INDEX

263

SUBJECT INDEX

A

Acoustical phonetician, 100
Affricatives, 210
Allophones
variations in, 8-11
anticipatory coarticulation, 10-11
coarticulation, 9-10
syllable organization, 11
vowel reduction, 9
Alpha motoneuron, 31
Alveolar consonants, 6
American Speech and Hearing Association, 24, 168
Antecedent events, 139, 141-143
Articular system, 32
Articulation behavior, 107
learned, 235
skilled and unskilled, 238
Articulation, developmental aspects
babbling, 53, 54
competition of responses, 93
contraction theory, 54
distinctive stimulus, 94
expansion theory, 54
importance of babbling, 55, 56
learning sounds not part of the language, 98-99
longitudinal study of, 72-79
mimicry theory, 261
prediction research, 65-66
response acquisition, 97-98
response association, 98
retention of responses, 94-97
transfer and competition, 98-104
Articulation diagnostics, 195-216
see Articulation measurement
behavioral evaluation, 195-200
first evaluation session, 196
generalization patterns, 213-216
item analysis, 205

multiple elicitation of responses, 197-198
Articulation, manner of, 14-18, 61
glottis, 16
laryngeal pitch control, 14
larynx, 15-18
pharyngeal action, 18
timing variations, 16-18
voicing, 18
Articulation measurement
auditory discrimination, 196, 200, 251
Deep Test of Articulation, 225
distortion concept rejected, 205
imitative tests, 196
in phonetic contexts, 196
inter-session, 202-204
intra-session, 201-202
in linguistic contexts, 197
Properant, 107
Screening Deep Test, 173, 179, 185, 191
spontaneous picture tests, 196
Templin-Darley Test of Articulation, 59, 118, 123, 173
testing, 195-216
Triota Screening Battery, 173
Articulation, place of, 5-15
Articulation system, 27
Articulation therapy
aids in prognosis, 136
automated, 109-136
behavioral,
see Articulatory modification by behavioristic methods; Articulatory modification by the paired-stimuli technique; Articulatory modification through an ecletic approach
cost effectiveness of, 130-132
ear training, 196, 251
eclectic approaches to, 233-262

267